American Medical Association
Physicians dedicated to the health of America

D0746459

EHR

Implementation

Carolyn P. Hartley
Edward D. Jones, III

Foreword by Newt Gingrich
Founder, The Center for Health Transformation
Author, *Saving Lives & Saving Money*

AMA *press*

A Step-by-Step Guide for the Medical Practice

AMA Press

Vice President, Business Products: Anthony J. Frankos
Publisher: Michael Desposito
Director, Production and Manufacturing: Jean Roberts
Senior Acquisitions Editor: Marsha Mildred
Developmental Editor: Katharine Dvorak
Copy Editor: Mary Kay Kozyra
Director, Marketing: J. D. Kinney
Marketing Manager: Erin Kalitowski
Senior Production Coordinator: Boon Ai Tan
Senior Print Coordinator: Ronnie Summers

Additional copies of this book may be ordered by calling 800 621-8335 or from the secure AMA Press Web site at www.amapress.org. Refer to product number OP322205.

ISBN 1-57947-643-0

Library of Congress Cataloging-in-Publication Data

Hartley, Carolyn P.
 EHR implementation : a step-by-step guide for the medical practice / Carolyn P. Hartley, Edward D. Jones, III ; foreword by Newt Gingrich.
  p. ; cm.
 Summary: "A how-to-guide to the process of researching, selecting, negotiating, and implementing an electronic health record"—Provided by publisher.
 Includes bibliographical references and index.
 ISBN 1-57947-643-0
 1. Medical records—Data processing. 2. Medical offices—Management.
[DNLM: 1. Medical Records Systems, Computerized. 2. Automatic Data Processing. 3. Practice Management, Medical—methods. W 80 H3318e 2005] I. Title: Electronic health records implementation. II. Jones, Ed (Edward Douglass) III. Title.

 R864.H375 2005
 610'.285—dc22   2004025326

BP02:04-P-046:02/05

To Michyla Grace and Logan James, who will grow up using EHRs as if there were never any other way to manage a health record, and to their family members, who will learn from the children how to use them.

FOREWORD

Fifteen years ago, debit cards were still a novelty. Now, there are more debit cards in America than there are Americans. ATMs outnumber bank branches four to one. Society's reliance on this technology has become so pervasive that consumers rank ATM/debit cards as the number two most important item in their lifestyles immediately behind the home phone—beating out computers, cell phones, internet, and cable TV. An American bank that does not offer customers 24-hour access to their bank account through an ATM will not be in banking very long.

Ten years ago, airline electronic ticketing was still considered the alternative way to travel. Now, 90% of consumers use e-ticketing, and airlines are charging as much as $50 more for paper tickets. The International Air Transport Association set a goal of eliminating paper ticketing worldwide by 2007. I speak to audiences all over the country about health transformation and when I ask the audiences if they used an e-ticket to get to the conference, 95% of the hands go up.

Jeffrey D. Cooper, MD, owns a one-site solo pediatric practice in Duluth, Georgia. He used a workflow-designed electronic health record (EHR) system to increase the number of children the office can serve from 10,000 to 15,000 with no staff increase. Only 12 of his two-year-old patients lack the appropriate vaccines because the system automatically reminds the staff when a child is due for a vaccine. The team at Cooper Pediatrics is practicing better medicine with less red tape with increased revenue.

In less than ten years, EHR will be as ubiquitous as ATMs and e-ticketing. Purchasing EHRs and the infrastructure to support them will be as fundamental as budgeting for examination tables, telephones, and stethoscopes. Why am I so confident? Because health is more important than air travel and banking and yet these industries have already moved to electronic systems; because paper medical records and paper prescriptions are killing patients and our society will simply no longer tolerate it; because the benefits of an interconnected healthcare system are growing increasingly more evident, which will transform EHR from a novelty to a necessity.

America needs a medical system that uses interoperable EHRs.

We need EHRs to save lives.

We need EHRs to prevent needless suffering.

We need EHRs to make our healthcare system affordable.

We need EHRs to help solve the growing physician and nurse shortage by freeing up medical talent from time consuming administrative tasks.

We need EHRs to return medicine to a system that attracts the best and the brightest young people to the profession.

We need EHRs to create a virtual public health and biosurveillance system.

We need EHRs to help accelerate research and discovery.

We need EHRs to help support the establishment of a new system of medical justice.

We need EHRs to make it easier for individuals to learn about and become engaged in their healthcare.

The medical profession needs interoperable EHRs.

You need an EHR to practice the best medicine possible.

You need an EHR to decrease your operational and administrative costs and increase your take-home pay.

You need an EHR to help in the prevention of costly and harmful medical mistakes.

You need an EHR to help reduce your risk of and defend against medical malpractice lawsuits.

You need an EHR to optimize your resources and the talent of your team.

You need an EHR to compete in the growing transparent consumer-driven market system where patients are being incentivized to choose doctors based on quality of care and/or use of information systems.

You need an EHR to easily demonstrate positive outcomes that qualify you for the increasing number of pay-for-performance program bonuses.

You need an EHR to easily share vital medical information with your patients that will help them to take more responsibility for their care.

You need an EHR to allow you to spend more time doing what you went into medicine to do—help patients.

If you are beginning this book dubious of the varied and impressive benefits of EHRs, you won't be after you finish reading the countless real-life implementation examples Carolyn and Ed have assembled. If you are confused about how to successfully chose, purchase, and execute an EHR in your medical practice, you won't be after you finish reading.

If you work in an office or care facility that is still using paper medical records, paper prescription pads, and paper lab orders, you need to read this book. *EHR Implementation: A Step-by-Step Guide for the Medical Practice* is your tool-kit for realizing the most significant contribution your medical generation can make to history—fundamentally altering the practice of medicine by adopting interoperable EHRs and maximizing their potential.

Newt Gingrich
Founder, The Center for Health Transformation
Author, *Saving Lives & Saving Money*
Speaker of the US House of Representatives, 1995–1999

PREFACE

Electronic health records (EHRs) have been poised to be a successful and innovative technology since the early 1980s. For the last 10 years, distinguished health care policy leaders, along with members of Congress and information technology influencers, have launched an expansive public affairs campaign to educate consumers on the need for health information transformation.

There was a tremendous upsurge in the campaign in 2004, which came on the heels of several pivotal actions: The RAND study, *Profiling the Quality of Care in Twelve Communities: Results From the CQI Study,*[1] was the largest and most comprehensive examination ever conducted of health care quality in the United States. The report revealed that people across the country were at risk for receiving poor health care. In addition, the Institute of Medicine announced its national priority areas and, in Executive Order 13335, President Bush appointed David J. Brailer, MD, PhD, to be the National Health Information Technology Coordinator.

In short, the cards are stacked; the writing is on the wall; consumers are now on board the health care transformation train. It's time for everyone to get an electronic medical record (EMR).

By 2008, it will be difficult to tell patients that your office isn't equipped to read or update their EHR. An explanation may be quaint and defendable, but risky. A practice telling a patient "Sorry, but we do not use EHRs" would be like a bank having to inform customers that they can't access the bank's automated teller machine (ATM) or conduct online banking.

An EMR allows patients to be immediately involved in health care decisions and care management. More than ever, patients want a relationship with their doctor. They also want to feel special enough to get in and out of the office in a timely fashion and back to being healthy and productive. A 2-hour wait is not acceptable, nor is it necessary. The patient immediately benefits from EHRs, but your practice is where it all begins.

The decision to automate will alter your workforce's administrative and clinical duties and it will affect office culture. Get buy-in from everyone who will be affected, including administrative and clinical workforce members. An office with a well-defined workflow runs like a well-oiled machine, freeing physicians and administrators from thinking about day-to-day operations.

The rewards may seem obscure at first. But they are there. Truth be told, a primary force driving physicians to EMRs is the fact that physicians need data to make clinical decisions about patient care, to spend more time in patient care, to get reimbursed accurately and on time, to receive bonuses from employers who want healthy employees, and to reduce malpractice insurance rates.

Regardless of where you are in the electronic health information process, *EHR Implementation: A Step-by-Step Guide for the Medical Practice* is for you. You may learn something new about the EMR system you've already purchased. If you're in the EHR system evaluation process, this book will be your guide.

You will learn how to evaluate and map out your workflow—a critical process that will help you select the EHR system that's right for your practice. Show your workflow charts to the EMR system vendors so that they can customize the software for you, which is a much better scenario than having software that has been customized for other practices. You'll also follow a logical and well-defined selection process that describes each step, supported by a well-defined implementation process.

We visited more than 50 physician offices to learn what worked and what didn't work. We participated in vendor demonstrations and EHR implementation and training sessions so that this book would be a real-world guide for you.

We combed through thousands of pages of EHR standards documentation, making it possible for you to review and comment on the EHRs that are in testing and revision stages with health standards organizations. With EHR standards at the stage of "draft standards for trial use" (DSTU), you still have time to influence how they will function in the physician's practice. You helped shape the outcome of the Health Insurance Portability and Accountability Act of 1996 (HIPAA) Security Rule and made it easier to implement. This book will show you how you can shape the outcome of EHRs.

How to Use This Book

You'll want a highlighter, a pen, and a notepad at your side when you read this book. It is a working document filled with flowcharts, graphs, checklists, and clear implementation steps to help you research, select, negotiate, and implement an EHR system in your medical practice.

Content is divided into two parts. Part 1 presents practical implementation steps to guide you through the EHR selection, purchase, and implementation stages. Part 2 is for those who want the details of how an EHR functions and how it will impact your return on investment. We identify the specific functions of each EHR standard in narrative format. As you review each standard, you can identify those that are useful in your practice now, as well as standards that will bring you a positive return on investment.

Following is an overview of what you will find in each chapter.

Part 1: A Step-by-Step Guide Through the Selection, Purchase, and Implementation of Electronic Health Records

Chapter 1: The Basics of Electronic Medical Records and Electronic Health Records

This chapter provides an overview of the influences that are reshaping the quality of health care today, including the Institute of Medicine's report on priority areas for national action and the Framework for Strategic Action, which was designed by the Office of the National Coordinator for Health Information Technology. We explain the difference between EMRs, EHRs, and PHRs (personal health records) and what these electronic record systems should do for you and your practice. Finally, we present industry trends in adopting electronic record systems to help you forecast what you'll need in the next 5 to 10 years.

Chapter 2: Electronic Medical Records: Your Electronic Workflow Assistant in the Medical Office

This chapter is filled with charts that compare paper workflow to electronic workflow in a physician's office. A mini–EHR vendor demonstration is included so that you can see how administrative and clinical work flows when it is parlayed into an EMR environment. This chapter is a must for office managers and EHR physician champions who want a system that is highly functional in their specialty, rather than a one-size-fits-all EMR.

Chapter 3: Making the Purchase

This chapter guides you through the purchase process and helps you decide what's right for your budget, workflow, and the people in your practice. You'll learn how to budget for an EMR and how to design your implementation dream team, and you'll follow a 12-step process to select the right system for your organization. Critical documents include a request for proposal (RFP) created for a small to midsize physician practice and a score card to help you evaluate vendors by function, usability, and cost.

You'll also get negotiation tips from the founder of a market institution that facilitates group purchases and EHR implementation training and technical support, including how to include the patient in your EHR/EMR decision.

Chapter 4: Making the Switch From Paper to Electronic Medical Records

Implementation may take 6 weeks to 6 months, depending on physician specialty, vendor involvement, budgets, and workforce attitudes and acceptance.

In this chapter, we discuss how to plan and budget for EHR implementation and how to positively engage staff in technology adoption. We've included case studies from other practices that have made the move to EHRs.

Part 2: Standards Relevant to the Physician's Practice

Chapter 5: Clinical Data Set Standards for Providers

In this chapter, you'll learn why the federal government has taken a new approach to technology in the clinical sector of the health care industry. The Consolidated Health Informatics program and the role of standards organizations in developing these programs are explained. You'll also learn the role of HIPAA Administrative Simplification with regard to these new initiatives and what data element code sets are included in the clinical initiatives.

Chapter 6: Electronic Health Records Systems: The Health Level Seven Draft Standards for Trial Use

This chapter describes the functional standards defined by Health Level Seven (HL7) and provides physicians with an opportunity to determine whether the standard is applicable to their practice and whether the practice wishes to comment on the standard. Functional areas worthy of your evaluation include direct care, supportive functions, and the information infrastructure of EHR systems.

We hope *EHR Implementation: A Step-by-Step Guide for the Medical Practice* will be the most marked up, highlighted book in your practice. It isn't designed to be a paperweight or to gather dust in your library. It was created to be a useful, easy-to-understand reference tool that your practice's EHR implementation team will use every day. We wish you great success and hope to hear more about your implementation strategies.

Warm wishes,
Carolyn Hartley
Ed Jones

Endnotes

1. RAND Corporation. Profiling the quality of care in twelve communities: results from the CQI study. *Health Affairs.* 2004;23:247–256.

ACKNOWLEDGMENTS

If the transformation of our nation's largest billing system occurs with the same cooperation that we received in writing this book, the healthcare system is in very good hands. We received incomparable support from members of standards-setting and review organizations, the Office of the National Coordinator for Health Information Technology, the Center for Health Transformation, members of Congress, and electronic health record vendors. We asked more than a dozen of the top EHR vendors to share screenshots with us so that you could see what workflow looked like in an electronic environment. Seven of those vendors responded enthusiastically and provided us with prompt information critical to your success.

From Allscripts Healthcare Solutions, we'd like to thank Paul Peterson, Chris Dahlberg, and David Nuckols; from Cerner, thanks go to Lindsey Henry Moss and Terron Bruner; from IntegriMED and eClinicalWorks, our thanks go to Laura Nasipak and Traci Detchon; from A4 Health Systems, we are grateful to Ray McDonald and Jennifer Lewis; from SynaMed, thanks go to Christeen Kim; and from MedFusion, we're grateful to Steve Malik. We believe the willingness of these companies to share information is an indication of the support you will receive when you inquire into their services.

From Health Level Seven committees and leaders, we'd like to thank Karen Van Hentenryck and Wes Rishel for allowing us to modify EHR functions into a narrative format for physician use. We'd also like to thank Gary Davidson, MD, and Linda Fischetti, RN, MS, co-chairs of the HL7 EHR Workgroups, for providing valuable insights into the standards-setting process.

Very special thanks go to the more than 50 physicians and office managers whom we interviewed, but in particular, we'd like to thank Dr David Paul Adams, Dr Scott Conard, Dr Doug Holmes, Dr Jerry Bernstein, Dr Bill Davis, Kemal Erkan, and Dr Simon J. Samaha. Thanks also to William McHenry, a practice manager and founder of the Quality Healthcare Center, a management service organization (MSO) serving physicians throughout the Southeast.

From the Office of the National Coordinator for Health Information Technology, we're deeply grateful to David J. Brailer, MD, PhD, for taking time to explain details of the Framework for Strategic Action and to Missy Krasner for her public affairs leadership. From Gingrich Communications, we're grateful to Kathy Lubbers, and in particular to Newt Gingrich for his leadership in this information-rich industry.

To our friends at AMA Press, we express deep gratitude for giving us extra time so that we could include current information in this book. In particular, we thank Marsha Mildred, Katharine Dvorak, John Kinney, and Erin Kalitowski for working extra hours to get this book into your hands. The author and publishing teams had you in mind when we created this real-world EHR guidebook.

ABOUT THE AUTHORS

Carolyn P. Hartley is president and CEO of Physicians EHR, LLC, an organization that advises physicians on EHR selection, implementation, and technical support. She also is editor-in-chief and publisher of "The Physician's e-Health Report," a bimonthly publication that advises physicians on technology techniques. She is author team leader of more than a dozen technology and compliance books for health care provider organizations including the *Field Guide to HIPAA Implementation, HIPAA Policies and Procedures Desk Reference*, and *Handbook for HIPAA Security Implementation*, all published by AMA Press. She is co-author with Ed Jones of *HIPAA Plain & Simple; HIPAA Transactions: A Nontechnical Business Guide for Health Care;* and the forthcoming book, *A Guide to Implementing Electronic Health Records*. She holds a master's degree in liberal arts from Baker University and maintains professional credentials as a Certified Health Privacy Professional (CHP). Carolyn can be reached at carolyn@physiciansehr.com.

    Edward D. Jones, III is executive vice president and member of the Board of Directors of FisaCure, Inc, in Carrollton, Texas. FisaCure tailors cost-effective electronic solutions for reconciling remittance advice documentation with payments for services for its health plan and health care customers. Ed also is a contributing editor with Physicians EHR, LLC, and chair of the Workgroup for Electronic Data Interchange (WEDI), a not-for-profit association of more than 200 members, including providers, payers, employers, government organizations, and standards groups. WEDI's mission is to foster successful implementation of Administrative Simplification standards under the federal Health Insurance Portability and Accountability Act of 1996 (HIPAA). Until 1999, Ed served as senior vice president of The Centris Group, Inc, which comprised seven subsidiary companies with a core focus on underwriting and reinsuring self-funded plans for US employers.

    Ed holds degrees in economics from the University of Chicago and Washington University in St. Louis. He can be reached at ejones@fisacure.com.

CONTENTS

A Step-by-Step Guide Through the Selection, Purchase, and Implementation of Electronic Health Records

The Basics of Electronic Medical Records and Electronic Health Records

*The fragmentation of our healthcare system poses barriers to communication between hospitals and practices, and between practices and research facilities. With the push of a button, a doctor should be able to receive the latest scientific articles along with his patient's chart, or prescribe a medicine and send it to the pharmacy. But often, the systems are not in place for them to do so. These barriers to communication don't serve physicians, and they don't serve patients either. —**Senator Hillary Rodham Clinton**[1]*

Their politics aside, US senators from Bill Frist (R-TN) to Newt Gingrich (Center for Health Transformation) and Hillary Rodham Clinton (D-NY) all agree that the transformation of healthcare from paper to an electronic environment is very big stuff.

If you're like most physicians, you've read articles, white papers, and reports and you've heard present and former members of Congress hail the bright future of interoperable electronic health records (EHRs) that integrate a variety of clinical and administrative functions and information streams. Most likely, you've also researched a company or two that offers electronic medical records (EMRs) and talked to colleagues and vendors to evaluate what's best for your practice.

This chapter begins to define the differences between EHRs and EMRs and how they interrelate. We provide you with outlines of their basic functions, including charts, graphs, checklists, and trends, and offer a step-by-step outline for EMR implementation.

WHAT YOU WILL LEARN IN THIS CHAPTER

- The influences that are reshaping quality healthcare, including the Institute of Medicine report

- Physicians who are at the center of the movement toward the adoption of health information technology
- The difference between EMRs, EHRs, and PHRs
- What electronic record systems should do for you and your practice
- Industry trends on the adoption of electronic record systems

Key Terms

Clinical Records: The archival accounting of care services provided through formal healthcare providers and institutions.

Continuity of Care: The process by which the patient and the physician are cooperatively involved in ongoing healthcare management toward the goal of high-quality, cost-effective medical care.[2]

Electronic Health Record (EHR): A secure, real-time, interoperable point-of-care, patient-centric information resource for clinicians. The EHR aids clinicians' decision making by providing access to patient health record information where and when they need it and by incorporating evidence-based decision support. The EHR automates and streamlines the clinician's workflow, closing loops in communication and response that result in delays or gaps in care. The EHR also supports the collection of data for uses other than direct clinical care, such as billing, quality management, outcomes reporting, resource planning, and public health disease surveillance and reporting.[3]

Electronic Health Record (EHR) System: A set of components that form the mechanism by which patient records are created, used, stored, and retrieved. The EHR system includes people, data, rules and procedures, processing and storage devices (paper, pen, hardware, software), and communication and support facilities. It also includes longitudinal collection of electronic health information for and about persons; immediate electronic access to person- and population-level information by authorized (and only authorized) users; provision of knowledge and decision support that enhance the quality, safety, and efficiency of patient care; and support of efficient processes for healthcare delivery.

Electronic Medical Record (EMR): A computerized practice management system providing real-time data access and evaluation in medical care. Together with clinical workstations and clinical data repository technologies, the EMR provides the mechanism for longitudinal data storage and access. A motivation for healthcare providers to implement this technology derives from the need for medical outcome studies, more efficient care, speedier communication among providers, and easier management of health plans.[4]

Health Level Seven (HL7): One of several standards-developing organizations (SDOs) accredited by the American National Standards Institute (ANSI) that operate in the healthcare arena. Most SDOs produce standards (sometimes called specifications or protocols) for a particular healthcare domain such as pharmacy, medical devices, imaging, or insurance (claims processing) transactions. Health Level Seven's domain is clinical and administrative data.

Interoperability: The ability to exchange and use information (usually in a large heterogeneous network made up of several local area networks). Interoperable systems reflect the ability of software and hardware on multiple machines from multiple vendors to communicate.[5]

Personal Health Record (PHR): Individually held and controlled lifelong repositories of (1) all clinical encounters; (2) health promotion activities; (3) personally valued health monitoring parameters such as exercise, nutrition, and spiritual well-being; (4) decision support, risk management, and professional advice; (5) consumer-focused health information and education; (6) benefits and financial management resources; and (7) environmental exposure and community health monitoring information.[6]

INSTITUTE OF MEDICINE IDENTIFIES PRIORITY AREAS FOR NATIONAL ACTION

In 1996, the Institute of Medicine (IOM) launched a concerted, ongoing effort to assess and improve the nation's quality of care. In question was the "fallibility of human healthcare providers, managers, and leadership" functioning in a complex, technologically driven, compartmentalized healthcare system. The IOM's conclusion was that "the burden of harm conveyed by the collective impact of all of our healthcare quality problems is staggering."[7]

As a result of the 1996 study and subsequent report, *Crossing the Quality Chasm: A New Health System for the 21st Century*,[8] the IOM created the IOM Quality Initiative and brought together leaders from exemplary communities and national organizations to study and redesign a new work environment that would keep patients safe. Representatives from several organizations that have helped shape the business of healthcare studied the following:

- How the experiences of patients should be changed
- How teams of healthcare workers should interact
- How healthcare organizations can better design work and institute proactive error-reduction strategies
- How policy officials and healthcare purchasers can reshape health policy to create a safer healthcare system[9]

In an article in its Winter 2002 newsletter,[10] the IOM documented abbreviated results of key findings in its report, *Crossing the Quality Chasm*. In this article, the authors called for a design of new systems that "prevent, detect, and minimize hazards and the likelihood of error." They stated that they "want a system in which it is hard to make a mistake and easy to do the right thing."[10]

TABLE 1-1

Simple Rules for the 21st Century Healthcare System

Current Approach	New Rule
Care is based primarily on visits	Care is based on continuous healing relationships
Professional autonomy drives variability	Care is customized according to patient needs and values
Professionals control care	The patient is the source of control
Information is a record	Knowledge is shared and information flows freely
Decision making is based on training and experience	Decision making is evidence based
"Do no harm" is an individual responsibility	Safety is a system property
Secrecy is necessary	Transparency is necessary
The system reacts to needs	Needs are anticipated
Cost reduction is sought	Waste is continuously decreased
Preference is given to professional roles over the system	Cooperation among clinicians is a priority

Source: The Institute of Medicine.[8]

Healthcare organizations collaborating on the IOM Quality Initiative spelled out new initiatives in patient management. The report recapped a wide array of patient safety initiatives, including advice that "information technology must play a central role in the redesign of the healthcare system if a substantial improvement in quality and safety is to be achieved over the coming decade. The Internet has enormous potential to transform healthcare as it has nearly every other facet of society."[10]

Prior to the IOM study, EMRs were considered academic, forward thinking, and costly technology. But when the IOM study pronounced EMRs "an essential technology for healthcare,"[10] it became the change agent for many practices in healthcare and captured the attention of legislators, policymakers, patient advocates, physicians, and proactive vendors. The IOM's report included rules for physicians and healthcare organizations. Note that EMRs can help physicians achieve several of the rules outlined in Table 1-1.

HEALTH LEVEL SEVEN LEADS THE STANDARDIZATION PROCESS

Your EMR may be a beautiful piece of software with exciting features for its time, but unless your vendor is participating in the adoption of one *common* set of standards, your EMR may end up in a storage garage.

First know the difference between an electronic health record (EHR) and an electronic medical record (EMR), advised Linda Fischetti, RN, MS, co-chair of the Health Level Seven (HL7) EHR Workgroups. Health Level Seven is an organization that is creating standards that define how health *messaging* will be exchanged.[11] In its most basic form, an *EMR* is the practice management system that stores health information about the patient. An *EHR* is a data set of health information that can be packaged and routed to another location, such as a lab, a pharmacy, or another provider, to be opened and read. An *EHR system* is the entire package, including people, systems, data, rules and procedures, and communication support and facilities that allows you to exchange administrative and clinical information about a patient in a secure environment so that everyone involved in the patient's care has access to appropriate information when they need it.

The EHR process follows the same International Standards Organization (ISO) standards-setting process that allows you to purchase a Toyota or BMW and to get it serviced locally, even though it was manufactured overseas. The ISO standards in other industries give you the freedom to shop online, track the status of your overnight shipment, or withdraw money from your checking account from any bank's automated teller machine (ATM).

The HL7 *EHR-System Functional Model and Standards* was approved as a Draft Standard for Trial Use (DSTU) in July 2004. These draft standards will be in pilot testing until summer 2006. Adopting the model doesn't mean vendors will start incorporating every function of the model, according to Pat Wise, who represents the Healthcare Information and Management Systems Society (HIMSS) on the EHR Collaborative,[12] a multidisciplinary group of healthcare stakeholders working to refine the EHR model. "It helps provide a guideline. It helps provide a standard," Wise said. The EHR Collaborative has provided ambitious and engaging feedback on the HL7 EHR-System Functional Model and Standard.

Chapters 3 and 4 of this book provide more of the collaborative, regulatory, and technical details and functional descriptors that will be beneficial as you conduct electronic record systems discussions with vendors.

PHYSICIAN GROUPS ARE AT THE CENTER OF HEALTH INFORMATION TECHNOLOGY ADOPTION

"From digital hospitals to sprawling physician groups, electronic medical records are moving from pipe dream to mainstream. But most MDs practice in small groups, and, as they embrace EMRs, their requirements will reshape a market. . . ," writes Eric G. Brown in a December 2003 Forrester Research report.[13]

Brown's conclusion is based on research findings from Forrester, an independent technology research company. The Forrester research findings predict that "EMR sales to physician practices will increase from $816 million in 2003 to $1.4 billion in 2008. In the same time period, spending will more than double among small physician practices, from $366 million to $829 million. By next year [2005], Forrester analysts say, for the first time, sales to small practices will surpass those to larger practices."[14]

Until now, vendor survival has been based on an EMR sales approach focused on large physician groups and hospital networks. That's where the money has been. A multimillion dollar sale to a hospital, even when the EMR is scaled down, can cost a small physician group the equivalent of months of practice revenue. And if the EMR provider goes belly-up, the physician's practice may not recover.

While vendors have focused on hospitals and large physician networks, the Forrester research indicates that 400,000 practicing physicians work in groups of eight or fewer, and it's the smaller groups that are driving EMR developers to consider a new marketing—and development—approach.

But now, there is good news for smaller physician groups. Costs are going down. Healthcare stakeholders are generally moving toward agreement on what electronic record systems should do for a healthcare provider in terms of handling clinical and administrative data and incorporating communication protocols. And vendor and provider experiences with EMRs are going to make it easier for physicians to calculate their returns on investment in EHR systems.

A Physician Leads Health Information Technology Adoption

"The physician-patient relationship should be the focus of healthcare reform from the inside out," said David J. Brailer, MD, PhD. "Encouraging physicians to integrate technology into their practices will be crucial to hospitals successfully computerizing their own systems."[15]

In Executive Order 13335, President George W. Bush named Dr Brailer to be the national health information technology (HIT) coordinator effective May 6, 2004.[16] His task is to provide leadership for reaching the 10-year goal of deploying electronic health records throughout the US healthcare system. He is charged with facilitating the vision for most Americans to have a personal health record by 2014. Some say it will happen long before then.

Of importance to physicians is that Dr Brailer has put a strong emphasis on physician adoption of technology. "HIT is not about computerization," Dr Brailer wrote in *Use and Adoption of Computer-based Patient Records*, a report prepared for the California Healthcare Foundation.[17] "It's about what we do with information and changing concepts of care so that information is seen as a form of therapy. Healthcare IT needs to allow for interconnectivity from one system to another and provide for the needs of population-based healthcare," Brailer wrote. "The lack of interoperability has been a barrier to physician adoption." It raises the risk of selecting the wrong system, he added, because without interoperability a physician's ability to choose an alternative system is constrained. The data itself must be mobile, down to the individual patient. "To me, this is fundamental," Brailer said.

National Health Information Technology Plan From the Department of Health and Human Services

In rolling out his national HIT plan, Dr Brailer laid out in the Framework for Strategic Action Progress Report a three-phase plan that will benefit providers and hopefully stabilize the price of EHR systems.[18]

Phase I of the plan focuses on the development of market institutions. Examples of market institutions are certification organizations, group purchasing entities, and low-cost implementation support organizations. "They [market institutions] will lower the risk of HIT procurement, thereby enhancing demand and making more efficient use of resources that are invested. They will enhance the depth and confidence of HIT buyers and will accelerate the introduction of quality and efficiency into the mainstream of care delivery," Brailer explained.

Phase II involves investment in clinical management tools and capabilities based on substantial savings as EHR systems become certified. Phase III will transition the market to robust quality and performance accountability (quality and clinical performance monitoring linked to public reporting and incentive reimbursements).

When it comes to low-cost EHR partnerships, watch for the application from the Veterans Administration (VA), which was made available for free to physicians in November 2004. Its use, however, may be more applicable to long-term care and rehabilitation facilities than to the physician practice.

As a follow-up to the Framework for Strategic Action Progress Report, 14 physician associations announced their participation in the Physicians EHR Coalition. Since its creation, membership has expanded to 20 physician associations. The following news release, housed at several association Web sites, including the American Academy of Family Physicians, announces the formation of the Physicians Electronic Health Record Coalition (PEHRC)[19]:

> Fourteen preeminent medical organizations, representing more than 500,000 US physicians, announced the creation of the Physicians Electronic Health Record Coalition (PEHRC) today. This groundbreaking healthcare coalition will assist

physicians, particularly those in small- and medium-size ambulatory care medical practices, to acquire and use affordable, standards-based EHR systems and other HIT to improve quality, enhance patient safety and increase efficiency.

The acronym of QUALITY defines the PEHRC's guiding principles:

Quality
Usability
Affordability
Long-term commitment
Interoperability
Trust (Data stewardship, financial stability, integrity)
Yield (Work must provide tangible benefits for physicians)

The PEHRC is committed to taking practical steps to educate physicians about the value and best use of EHRs, to assist doctors in selection of systems, and to help focus the market on high quality and affordable products. Additionally, the PEHRC will work to participate in the development of the EHR certification process.

A representative from the Office of the National Coordinator for Health Information Technology said that the office hopes PEHRC will represent the voice of physicians in defining market institutions, creating a vendor certification structure, educating patients, and helping to stabilize the cost of EHRs.[20]

Patients Await Electronic Health Record Technology

Even though patients were given the right to view their own medical records when the Health Insurance Portability and Accountability Act of 1996 (HIPAA) Privacy Rule went into effect in April 2003, few have bothered. The hassle to visit the doctor's office, fill out paperwork, and wait for 30 days has been daunting. But EHRs will give patients a faster look.

Dr Chen-Tan Lin, senior medical director of informatics at the University of Colorado Health Sciences Center (UCHSC), said that although 80% to 90% of patients would like to see their medical records, less than 1% have actually done so.[21] However, a report by that university indicates that if given a chance, patients want electronic access to those health records.

By June 2004, patients at the UCHSC who had access to EHRs were able to monitor their cholesterol levels, download low-sodium diet information, and send questions via e-mail to their doctors. Doctors did not filter the information that patients were able to access from their records. The university's electronic medical system allows patients to access key parts of their medical histories, including lab results, doctors' notes, x-rays, and medications.

THE DIFFERENCE BETWEEN ELECTRONIC MEDICAL RECORDS, ELECTRONIC HEALTH RECORDS, AND PERSONAL HEALTH RECORDS

For more than a decade, the healthcare industry has struggled not only with technology adoption, but also with how to define EMRs. The technology behind EMRs is mature, but campaigns on what to call them needed clarification, definition, and acceptance.

To date, the healthcare industry has assigned at least 13 sets of terminologies and definitions for EMRs.[17] Most of those terms have arisen from vendor marketing efforts to claim "mind share" over what EMRs should actually be called.

One term that gained popularity was *computer-based patient record* (CPR) because the name closely defined itself to consumers. But even among the CPR audience, "there was disagreement about what functions should be considered part of a CPR."[17] The more commonly used term today is *personal health record* or PHR.

The Electronic Medical Record

To physicians and healthcare providers, the term *electronic medical record* (EMR) makes sense because it refers to the electronic version of the paper records created in most physician offices. In its simplest form, an EMR is the software that houses confidential patient information in an electronic format, quite similar to what the filing cabinet has done for paper records over the last 150 years. Unlike its paper siblings, the EMR offers search capabilities, makes electronic records easy to locate and read, takes up little office space, and eliminates significant administrative costs. It also can be transported in a wireless environment so that records can be accessed from remote locations.

Upon command, an EMR can generate a summary of a patient's contact information, including name, address, date of birth, insurance information; clinical data, such as a summary of the patient's medical history, documentation of each encounter, symptoms, diagnosis, treatment, and outcome; and medical error and coding cross references, such as a history of allergies and adverse reactions; and it cross-checks allowable codes, which prevents billing errors. An EMR can also provide you with valuable demographic information, such as:

- Zip codes where the majority of your patients live
- Identification of payers that are most profitable
- Medical conditions that you treat most frequently
- Physicians who most frequently refer patients to you

An EMR is usually created and licensed by a software vendor, and in today's entrepreneurial market, the EMR may result from a combination of several companies working together.[22] These electronic relationships present privacy and security concerns, which is why the Department of Health and Human Services (HHS) imposed privacy and security rules as a foundation for EMR confidentiality and electronic use. With privacy and security in place, physicians and patients can have greater confidence when using and disclosing electronic health information.

Privacy and Security First

Although an EMR as a software application is not regulated by HHS, the manner in which health information is electronically created, stored, and transmitted is regulated by the Administrative Simplification standards regulations pertaining to HIPAA Transactions and Code Sets and its Privacy and Security Rules.[23]

Before you implement an EMR in your practice, your privacy and security officials must ensure that the use, disclosure, and electronic transfer of patient records will be conducted in a confidential, secure environment.

The Electronic Health Record

The biggest difference between an EMR and an EHR is this: the EHR includes the technology that moves the patient's record from one place to another. An EMR is the staging platform, or file cabinet, that contains the EHR. Electronic health records are a more complex version of an EMR and fundamentally depend upon interoperability or communication among and between multiple healthcare stakeholders.

For a patient, an EHR is like having the entire clinical, research, educational, and administrative team of researchers, caregivers, insurers, and thought leaders gather in one room to review, share, and discuss the latest diagnostic and treatment plans, avoid duplication of tests, agree upon successful coding and payment strategies, and determine what's in the best interest of the patient.

For a physician, an EHR is an immediate, reliable, and searchable database that is used to make therapeutic decisions for the best clinical outcomes. The EHR allows the physician to:

- Integrate data from multiple sources
- Capture data at the point of care
- Offer clinical support in decision making

Figure 1-1 illustrates how information flows into an EHR.

The Personal Health Record

The personal health record (PHR) contains medical information and it is owned by the patient. Information contained in the PHR may have been created by any number of sources including the patient, a lab, a

FIGURE 1-1

Data Sources for the EHR

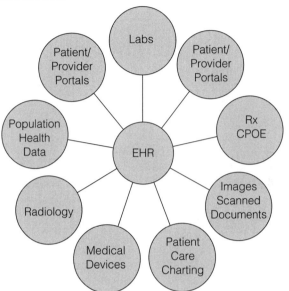

Rx CPOE indicates computerized physician order entry (for prescriptions); EHR, electronic health record.

physician's practice, a hospital, an organ transplant organization, or an insurance company.

An example of an early PHR is a bracelet that contains vital health information about a patient. For example, a patient with internal titanium parts from reconstructive orthopedic surgery may need a PHR bracelet to get through airport-security metal detectors. Or, a patient with diabetes may wear a bracelet so that an emergency physician will know how best to administer treatment if the patient goes into a diabetic coma.

Developers of PHR technology will exponentially proliferate as EHRs become interoperable and as physicians adopt EMRs as the standard format for maintaining patient records. Some PHR software developers are collaborating in the standardization process so that the patient's PHR can be used, read, and updated by multiple providers. An example of how PHR technology may be used in clinical practice is in the following scenario:

A patient comes into your office with the PHR on a memory stick or thumb drive that contains the patient's medical records.[24] That PHR likely contains the medical and personal history that the patient wants you to know, such as name, address, photo ID, insurance information including co-pay, eligibilities and required authorizations, chronic diseases, blood type, prescriptions, allergies, adverse reactions, emergency data, and family contact information. If your practice has been referred by another physician, the PHR likely contains information on earlier encounters. Ideally, the PHR contains data that are compatible with your system.

After examination, you might send the patient to a lab for tests. The lab technician performs requested tests and then downloads the results onto the memory stick. The patient brings the memory stick back to your office for immediate interpretation of the results, or the lab may send test results directly to you so that you and the patient can discuss the results.

You can see immediate benefits and challenges to both the patient and physician's office. Benefits include:

- Immediate access to health information, including lab results
- Reduced duplication of records
- Improved patient safety
- Improved workflow
- Greater patient responsibility for healthcare

Presently, most healthcare providers are excited if they can access just some of a patient's information electronically. The challenge in this high level of interoperability is how to make the EHR/EMR/PHR information compatible across communication protocols and electronic systems. Other industries have done it. Now, it's healthcare's turn to thrive.

In Figure 1-2 you can see how the patient's health record needs to be in sync with the records maintained by the physician.

THE ELECTRONIC MEDICAL RECORD AND THE ELECTRONIC HEALTH RECORD AS STANDARD REFERENCES

The HHS is most interested in how the EHR is developed, exchanged, used in decision making, and made available for provider and patient involvement. By 2014, HHS intends for EHRs to be used by patients, hospitals, laboratories, public health entities, and other healthcare stakeholder systems to communicate using one standard format.

Therefore, for the remainder of this book, the term *EMR* will refer to information software tools (electronic filing cabinets) used by the physician's office or other healthcare provider, and *EHR* will refer to an electronic software data file that electronically stores and transports standardized patient health information from one healthcare provider to another and is accessible (and usable) by providers. The PHR is owned and maintained by the patient. (Details about the process to standardize EHR formats, its testing in draft stage, and final adoption process are discussed in Part II of this book in Chapters 5 and 6. Details on EMR purchasing decisions are discussed in this chapter and Chapter 3.)

FIGURE 1-2

An EHR Is Patient-Focused; an EMR Is Physician-Focused

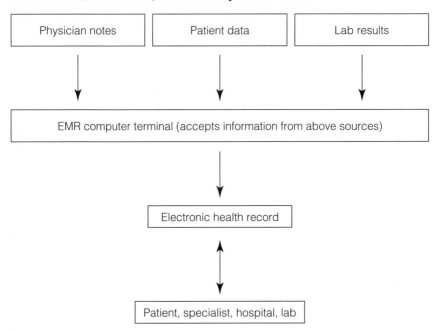

EMR indicates electronic medical record.

THE MOVE TO INTEROPERABILITY

In order to make an EHR interoperable and transportable, healthcare providers, including physicians, hospitals, pharmacies, and other providers, must evaluate software that enables health information to be read, edited, transmitted, received, and understood.

Physicians are no longer pondering *whether* to purchase EHR-compatible software but *what* to purchase. Purchasing questions regarding technology adoption now are more thought-provoking and budget driven and often involve significant technology, work flow and culture changes in the physician's practice:

- What should I buy?
- Will I need new computers?
- Is it too early to purchase software? Will prices continue to drop?
- How will EMRs change in the next two to five years?
- How long will it take my staff to learn how to use it?
- How much will it cost? Will it be less expensive two years from now?

■ How soon will I receive a return on investment?

■ Will my vendor be around two years from now when EHR standard formats become effective?

By the time you finish reading this book, you'll know the answers to these questions.

WHAT AN ELECTRONIC MEDICAL RECORD SHOULD DO FOR YOU AND YOUR PRACTICE

First and foremost, an EMR should be like a highly intelligent robotic employee that significantly reduces administrative tasks, especially unproductive and costly workflow processes. It should keep an accurate health record on each patient so that you don't have to search for a paper file and flip through pages. It also should act like a colleague who reviews clinical evidence when you need decision support.

Every provider, coder, manager, and patient knows that quite a bit of administrative time is spent sorting, searching, retrieving, issuing, and recovering medical records. An EMR won't take the place of an office manager but it will give the office manager dependable support.

An EMR doesn't require vacation time; it doesn't get sick, and it doesn't misplace records. It will, however:

■ File and retrieve records when you ask it to

■ Let you know if a drug can cause an adverse reaction

■ Remind you of patient allergies

■ Notify your patients when they should come in for routine exams

■ Identify potential billing errors to avoid rejected claims

■ Notify you when a deposit should be made into your account

It also provides a clinical template that you can customize for each patient, eliminating transcription costs. In the following sections are examples of what an EMR can do for you and your practice.

Reduce Administrative Burdens

It's no secret that physicians and staff are burdened with administrative challenges, constantly feeling the squeeze to see more patients, pay higher malpractice premiums, maintain accurate documentation on each patient, keep up with medical breakthroughs, protect patient confidentiality, get reimbursed less, and maintain a pleasant work environment.

Small wonder that a 2004 Merritt Hawkins report indicated that 76% of physicians between the ages of 50 and 65 found the practice of medicine to be less satisfying in 2004 than five years ago and that 51% of that same physician group intended to make a career change in the next three to five years. But that same group also said that patient relationships represented 58% of the greatest source of professional satisfaction.[25]

So an EMR that manages the majority of the practice's administrative burdens, while it reduces medical errors, provides codes that reduce denied claims, and directly stabilizes or reduces malpractice rates, could look attractive.

File, Retrieve, and Sort Medical Records

Jeff Johnson, MD, an internist at the Central Utah Multi-Specialty Clinic said that he has reduced by 35% to 40% the time his staff spends searching for patient charts (10 to 15 minutes per chart). "I didn't hire my nurses to do paper work," he said.

The practice, which includes nine locations and 59 physicians with 13 subspecialties, schedules between 450 and 500 daily patient visits with approximately 350 to 400 walk-ins and phone calls each day that require staff to pull additional charts. He said that the practice's chart room with 200,000 charts, including 130,000 active charts, no longer could contain the volume, which had spilled over into the practice's conference room.[26]

In the practice's paper-based office, Dr Johnson remembers turning around patient records in 3 weeks. Sometimes nurses would create shadow charts and keep information at their desks up to a month. But with the adoption of an EMR from Allscripts Healthcare Solutions (www.allscripts.com), physicians in this practice are turning records within 24 hours.

Gather and Help Analyze Data

In healthcare, data equals dollars. And managing data electronically equals even more dollars. Phase III of Dr Brailer's Framework for Strategic Action "transitions the market to robust quality and performance accountability. In this phase, clinicians will have the tools and capabilities to manage patients and populations, and to deliver consistently high-quality care in an efficient manner."[18]

Health plans and self-insured employers have started offering bonus programs for physicians who document quality. For example, the Bridges to Excellence program, which includes General Electric, Procter and Gamble, Ford Motor, Verizon Communications, and United Parcel Service, is available to physicians in Albany, Boston, Louisville, and Cincinnati.

"To qualify, doctors must demonstrate that they have implemented certain care management systems. Participating doctors will receive an annual $50 per-patient bonus, which is about half of the projected savings from the technology, according to the Bridges program. The program estimates that savings from these IT systems are about 4% to 5% of total care costs."[27]

A good EMR application should help you compile and analyze data about the quality of care your practice provides, sources of patient referrals, and your best payer relationships. In addition, it should help you identify and retrieve data you'd like to use to evaluate your practice's operations. Most important, it should help you identify and evaluate data on patient care, quality of services delivered to patients, patient outcomes, and costs.

In an era of chemical weapons and epidemics of infectious diseases, the types of data mining outlined above also can safeguard and advance the health of the patient population of your practice and provide benefits to your community as well.

Improve the Prescription Process

Doug Holmes, MD, an ear, nose, and throat (ENT) specialist in Raleigh, North Carolina, said the process to refill a prescription using paper records involved more than 10 steps, each involving human action. Using the EMR he purchased from Misys Healthcare Systems (www.misyshealthcare.com), he has reduced the task to three steps, all of them trackable on the computer.

When a patient calls in for a refill, the nurse sends an electronic message to the physician. Linked to the message is the patient's record. The physician can either choose to electronically fax the refill to the pharmacy, in which case the refill is added to the patient's record, or send a message back to the nurse with additional care instructions.

Some EMRs may not yet contain computerized physician order entry (CPOE) features, but your software vendor should give you an idea of when those features will be available for your practice.

By January 2006, the Centers for Medicare and Medicaid Services (CMS) will begin offering prescription benefits to seniors and people living with disabilities with a prescription drug benefit.[28] This benefit, provided for in the Medicare Modernization Act of 2003 (MMA), covers about 41 million beneficiaries. Given that 91% of Medicare recipients fill at least one prescription per year,[29] it makes sense to CMS to automate the prescription process, which is one of the reasons that electronic prescriptions, or *e-prescribing*, generate high interest among physicians and medical societies.

E-prescribing can be stand-alone software, or it can be a function of an EMR. If your office performs multiple prescription renewals for patients and you regularly prescribe medications, e-prescribing software may be your best introduction to health information technology. A primary care provider may fall into this category. However, if you are a multi-specialty practice dependent on lab tests, hospital medical files and complicated billing systems, you are likely to be a better fit for an EHR.

Check Billing Codes to Reduce Rejected Claims

William Davis, MD, chief medical information officer of Winona Health and chief financial officer and partner in Family Medicine of Winona, Pennsylvania, said that when his family medical practice implemented an

EMR from Cerner Corporation (www.cerner.com) the practice showed remarkably improved revenues from automated documentation and coding.

"The EMR allowed us to accurately capture services through improved documentation and coding," Dr Davis said. "We aren't seeing any more patients than in prior years, but we showed a gross increase of $500,000 in the first year."[30]

Reduce or Eliminate Transcription Fees

Physicians spend an average of 1.5 hours a day documenting approximately 20 to 30 patient encounters, or the equivalent of 7 to 8 hours per week. This is the equivalent of 9 weeks per year that a physician and other providers spend documenting care for the year. Approximately 80% of that documentation is a repetition of normal findings.[31]

Dr Holmes, the Raleigh, NC, ENT specialist, was an Air Force surgeon before joining a private practice in 1994. "I was shocked at how poorly the records system was set up," he said.[32]

He went from a fully computerized system with secure access to patient records to paper-based records where clinicians shared patient information on 3 × 5 cards. When a patient came into the office for a follow-up to a surgical procedure, Dr Holmes said that his staff would run "willy-nilly" trying to find the chart.

When he opened his own private practice with a pediatric specialty, he started looking at EMRs and, in particular, voice recognition systems to help gain immediate access to patient records and eliminate the $20,000 he spent each year in transcription fees. But voice recognition technology was still new, and he spent more time correcting inaccurate translations than if he'd dictated them for transcription. "For several reasons, we jumped in big with the Misys Healthcare Systems' EMR," Dr Holmes said. "We haven't used a transcription service since implementing the system."

Increase Patient Throughput

In Irving, Texas, Scott Conard, MD, wants patients to communicate with him through his online portal prior to coming into the office. According to Dr Conard, patients can go to the practice's Web site (www.tienahealth.com), click the MyDocOnline patient portal for the practice, and answer specific questions that provide him with clinical information.

"Sometimes when I respond to the patient, I can call in a prescription or make a referral so that they don't have to come into the office," Dr Conard explained. "But if I think I need to see the patient, I'll already have an online history of the specific episode and they can bypass preliminary information-gathering when they come into the office. When I have advanced knowledge of the symptoms, I can get them in and out of the office much quicker."

In Raleigh, when Dr Holmes sees patients for postoperative visits, he quickly calls up the medical file and has immediate access to his notes. His EMR also allows him to flag specific conditions that appeared during surgery or in a previous exam so that he doesn't have to flip through the pages hoping he won't miss something important. Often patients on a return checkup spend only 10 or 15 minutes in the office. With a pediatric ENT specialty, Dr Holmes said the parents appreciate the reduced time in the office.

Reflecting the increasing use of online communications between physicians and patients, the American Medical Association "recently announced a new code for online medical communications," and a number of payers are beginning to reimburse such communications.[33]

A New CPT® Code Lets You Get Reimbursed for Online Patient Evaluation

As of July 1, 2004, healthcare providers may get reimbursed when "evaluating and managing patient encounters" with an established patient via a secure communication network. Of particular interest to physicians with Internet sites is a new CPT® Category III code, 0074T.

"If you have a phone call with a patient and you hang up the phone, the words vanish, but with email, patients have a written reference," said Arthur Levin, MD, FAAP, pediatrician with Advanced Pediatrics in Beachwood, Ohio. Dr Levin uses Medem's Online Consultation.™ "Patient response has been very positive—people like having the option to e-mail me. As a pediatrician, it's usually family members and parents who email me which can save them a trip to the office. Online consultation allowed me to offer a tremendous level of depth regarding a problem, with far greater efficiency than an office setting typically offers," Dr Levin said. "A lot of pediatric care is free counseling, but online consultation lets me get paid."

Online consultation starts with getting a Web site up and running. Several companies, including Medem, will create a Web site for you online.

"Most physicians and staff want a little handholding to get their Web sites up and running," said Steve Malik, president and CEO of MedFusion, identified as the nation's leading provider of physician Web sites and secure patient-to-physician communication applications by the American Academy of Family Physicians. On April 30, 2004, MedFusion and AAFP announced an agreement that allows active AAFP active members to create free Web sites. Consult www.aafp.org or www.medusion.net for more information about that offer.

Under MedFusion's plan, the physician is paged when an email inquiry arrives so that the physician isn't repeatedly checking to see if an e-mail has arrived.

"While women continue to be the primary users of online consultation, more men are coming online seeking solutions to health issues they wouldn't ordinarily discuss in an office setting," Malik said.

Reimbursement Procedure

Category III codes, first introduced in 2002, are temporary codes used for emerging technology, services, and procedures. Data gathered in Category III codes will allow "physicians and other qualified healthcare professionals, insurers, health services researchers, and health policy experts to identify emerging technology, services, and procedures for clinical efficacy, utilization, and outcomes." In practical terms, physicians using CPT code 0074T will contribute to the widespread adoption of online patient communications.

"There's been a significant up tick in physician interest since release of this CPT code because online consultation gives physicians a competitive advantage," Malik said. This online service benefits patients and providers.

Benefits of Online Encounters	
Benefits to Patients	**Benefits to Providers**
• Improved healthcare—patients are more inclined to ask for help than self-medicate	• Improves physician-patient relationship
• Removes guesswork: "Should I call the doctor, or shouldn't I?"	• Relieves administrative tasks from patients calling for nonemergencies
• Patients with chronic conditions can regularly consult with physician or nurse	• Better disease management, reduced administrative costs
• Patients in rural areas receive care without long drives to office	• Physician can deliver care to patients challenged by distance
• Patients describe symptoms directly to the physician	• Patients provide specific details when prompted
• Patient comments are translated directly into medical record	• Physician can check patient history for drug interactions, managed care formularies, clinical guidelines
• Eliminates long waits in medical office	• Helps manage unscheduled patient visits
• Less in-office time if physician already knows symptoms	• Physician has patient history in hand before patient arrives; less time in office

Category III codes for 2004 were released on January 1, 2004, to give payers time to build a payment structure, a structure that is based on the payer's policies and not on a yearly fee schedule. The July 1 deadline to process payment is not fixed if a payer is prepared to begin reimbursing before then. Since this is a new and optional CPT code, it may be news to payers, so be sure to consult with them on their payment policies.

According to a May 14, 2004, article in *Health Data Management*, New York-based insurer Group Health, Inc, plans to reimburse physicians who perform online

continued

consultations with patients using software from communications vendor RelayHealth. Group Health expects to pay physicians $25 for nonemergency Web visits.

Before opening your Web site for virtual patient visits, review this checklist:

Online Medical Evaluation Reimbursement Checklist

_____   Are your HIPAA privacy policies and procedures in place?

_____   Has your Web site provider given you written assurance that this is a secure site?

_____   Have payers agreed to reimburse for this CPT code? (If not, you may wish to charge a credit card fee for the online medical visit until payers begin reimbursements [$30 to $35 is standard credit card fee].)

_____   Did the Web site vendor train your staff on how to use the online medical office features?

The following description will provide you with details about CPT code 0074T:

CPT Code 0074T Description

Online evaluation and management service, per encounter, provided by a physician, using the Internet or similar electronic communications network, in response to a patient's request, established patient.

Article reprinted with permission from the May/June 2004 issue of Physician's e-Health Report.[34]

Improve Patient Safety

"At least three times a day, I remind patients about an allergy or an adverse reaction because they have forgotten," said Dr William Davis of Winona Health. "Patients expect doctors to remember everything about their health records when they come in for treatment."

Most patients only see one or two physicians, but doctors see hundreds of patients every week, he explained, which is why he relies on the EMR to flag a problem or contraindication. He believes patients with EHRs will get more involved in their own healthcare, especially because they have access to personal health information.

In Winona, Minnesota, the health community lives in the shadow of Mayo Clinic in Rochester, just 40 miles away. The health community wanted to remain independent, yet they also wanted a single shared record accessible by physicians, specialists, the community hospital, home health, and long-term care. In working with Cerner Corporation, they built a system in which all providers can access the same health information on patients, an arrangement that reduces guesswork and supports patients with chronic conditions.

"The biggest improvement in patient safety is when the system flags a drug interaction or allergy," Dr Davis said. "And not just in one practice, but the information is available to all providers in Winona's health community."

Patient safety isn't just an American health issue. In Italy, the Instituto Nazionale Tumori developed a short questionnaire that patients receive on their mobile phones and fill out based on symptoms such as weight loss, shortness of breath, and sleep loss. This system helps physicians monitor patients with chronic conditions, rather than having them come into the office for monthly checkups.[35]

In a test of the system, all 97 participating cancer patients who attempted to fill out the questionnaire on their mobile phones were successful. The program gathers the results on a secure Web page to provide doctors with a summary of patients' symptoms. A flashing light appears next to patients' names if they have dramatic changes in symptoms, which helps physicians to prioritize their patients' needs.

Improve Patient Communication and Relationships

Dr Conard believes some patients wait until symptoms are out of hand before consulting a physician. In some cases, patients can't give up a half day of work to come into the office, or a mother with young children finds it difficult to bring several children into the office when one is ill.

Online consultation allows patients to make inquiries about their health, and it provides Dr Conard an opportunity to build relationships while creating a more complete medical history. In several physician offices, a nurse practitioner routinely checks e-mail messages from patients. MyDocOnline and Medfusion, both online patient communication vendors, can page a physician if necessary. Physician Support Group Inc, a management service organization in Raleigh, North Carolina, provides e-mail communication support for its physician members and either calls or faxes treatment updates to the physician.

In the spirit of lessons learned from the business sector, exercise caution about how available you make yourself to e-mail messages as they can dramatically affect productivity. To make e-mail messages work for you, assign one clinical person to check messages every two or three hours.

If you are setting up your own online patient communication system, include a disclaimer that protects you from an at-risk patient saying, "But, I sent you an e-mail!" Your attorney can provide you with the appropriate wording, such as, "If this is an emergency, contact 911 or go to the nearest hospital."

"Men, who traditionally don't consult a physician until the condition is severe, have used online consultation more than anticipated. They talk about conditions that they might not want to mention to a nurse in my office," he said.

Internet consultation was not a big factor in the mid-1990s, but the IOM report indicates the future of self-directed patients bent on sharing decisions with doctors. The IOM recommends physicians bring patients into the Internet communications loop, but first establish the guidelines for online consultation. This includes educating the patients in self-management of their conditions and providing them with educational material, particularly important for patients with chronic diseases.

Improve Workflow Management

When patients complain that they've been lost in the healthcare system, the real problem is that there isn't a defined and well-thought-out workflow plan. Most hospitals function with only a few variations in workflow, primarily because hospital workers are assigned to do specific jobs. But in a medical practice, workers perform multiple jobs and these jobs vary by practice, especially in specialty practices. For example, a cardiologist runs an office much differently than a urologist, and neither of them run their practice like a family physician. Job descriptions vary and sometimes "who does what" is a bit influenced by personalities.

Following are several examples in which workflow breaks down in the medical office:

- A new OB-GYN patient wants to schedule an appointment. → The scheduler doesn't enter this as a new patient. The workload from filling out new patient information forms, obtaining insurance eligibility, taking vitals, and developing a care management program backs up the office for nearly 2 hours.
- A patient calls in for a prescription refill. → The file clerk pulls the record and leaves it in a pile for the nurse to review and present to the doctor. → The medical file gets shuffled and is placed on another physician's desk.
- The physician requests lab tests. → Lab results are faxed to the office. → Lab results are filed in another patient's chart.

In most cases, workflow is a function of administrative processes. In an electronic environment, the chart can be reviewed or moved with a mouse click. (In Chapter 2, we discuss workflow management in a paper office. We also provide examples of how work is triggered when someone sees paper and how it is triggered in an electronic environment.)

Conduct Clinical Research

The American Academy of Pharmaceutical Physicians (www.aapp.org) is a professional organization that represents physicians who spend the majority of their professional time in matters related to pharmaceutical medicine. Participation in clinical trials has become a new revenue source for physician group practices. For physicians who engage in clinical research, registries, and clinical trial-related efforts, an EMR should be flexible enough to build a database for individual or multiple physician users. But be certain your privacy and security policies have been implemented before you launch this new career choice.

Provide Clinical Decision Support

Physicians generally function in an isolated setting. They make decisions about patient care but limit face-to-face time in order to meet managed care guidelines. However, physicians would like to know how other physicians are treating specific conditions or they may need data on a new epidemic and treatment plan.

A RAND Corporation study, the second installment of the largest and most comprehensive examination ever conducted of healthcare quality in the US, finds that people in all parts of the country are at risk for receiving poor healthcare.[36] "What we now know is that it really doesn't matter where you live—only about 50% of the time are you getting the recommended care," said lead study author Eve A. Kerr, MD, MPH, of the Veterans Affairs Ann Arbor Healthcare System and the University of Michigan. "The lack of community level variation in overall quality should serve as a wakeup call to all communities to examine their own quality of care and determine how they can do a better job."[36]

In the Forrester Research Report, *Electronic Medical Records: A Buyer's Guide for Small Physician Practices*, the authors identified EMRs for smaller practices that have not focused enough on building sophisticated clinical alerts into their systems. "Buyers should spend some initial bargaining chips on obtaining the vendor's help to set up the various alerts and reminders offered by the system."[37]

Enhance Practice Management Software for a Robust Collections Module

Inderpal Chabra, MD, a physician in New York City, had been using an applications service provider (ASP) model for several years to help him manage his practice. But he was toggling between two distinct software applications when conducting billing and collections and building his EMR platform.

When he began using a medical practice suite from SynaMed™ (www.synamed.com), he was able to integrate scheduling, billing, and coding capabilities into the clinical and business aspects of the medical practice. He generates data and records on any Internet-connected personal computer, laptop, tablet, or other enabled device. Correct coding initiatives, local medical review policies, and national coverage determinations are programmed into the system to provide safeguards in coding. The program streamlines his notes and makes them compliant with Current Procedural Terminology (CPT®) guidelines.[38]

Use Standard Language so That Health Records From Other Organizations Are Interoperable in One Electronic Health Record

"If everyone acquired an EMR today without data and messaging standards, we'd end up with 3,000 to 50,000 silos of information," said John Quinn, principal at Capgemini. Your EMR may be a beautiful piece of software with exciting features for its time, but unless your vendor is participating in the adoption of one common set of standards, your EMR may end up in a storage garage.

What Docs Want in an EMR

Every EMR company can deliver a return on investment analysis. If they don't, there's no need to spend time with them. But will your practice experience that return in 90 days, six months, or five years?

"Most physicians would be happy if they could just get lab tests in an electronic format that's compatible with their system," said Steven S. Lazarus, PhD, fellow of HIMSS, president of Boundary Information Group in Denver, and co-author of several books, including *Handbook for HIPAA Security Implementation* (AMA Press; 2004).

"If a device helps physicians do their job more efficiently, they'll take a look at it," Dr Lazarus said. "They won't adopt an EMR because it's for the national good. They have to ask, 'What's in it for me?'"

He said additional hot spots are:

- Keep me from going to jail for fraud
- Keep me from making medical errors
- Shorten my billing timelines
- Give me faster patient throughput
- Help me through a drug recall

A cardiology client of Dr Lazarus received a recall on a drug with potentially fatal consequences. Using the EMR, within one hour, the practice identified all patients using the drug. Within one week, the at-risk patients had been through the office and received other prescriptions.

"Right now, the biggest attraction to physicians is e-prescribing," Dr Lazarus said. "There are at least 10 administrative and clinical steps between the time a patient calls for a prescription refill and the prescription is finally filled. An EMR with e-prescribing capabilities can shorten that process to two or three steps using a mouse click."

Start with an "I Want" list:

I want . . .

- *To stop misfiling charts*
- *Patient information in the correct file*

- *To improve the prescription refill process*
- *To check documentation against codes used for billing*
- *To increase patient throughput*
- *Better workflow management*
- *To go home an hour earlier every day*
- *To have a better relationship with my patients*

When talking to vendors, Dr Lazarus said to make sure you ask this critical question: What assurance can you give me that you will convert my data in storage into EHR standards when those standards are adopted nationwide in three to four years?

"If you get a commitment, you should value it highly," he said. "You don't want to be sitting in your office three years from now doing this transition all over again."

Aritcle reprinted with permission from the May/June 2004 issue of Physician's e-Health Report.[39]

INDUSTRY TRENDS

In the 15th Annual HIMSS Leadership Survey sponsored by Superior Consultant Company,[40] Health Information Technology vendors were asked to provide information on what clients wanted from them now and two years from now. Patient safety and EMR implementation topped both lists.

Figures 1-3, 1-4, and 1-5 give you a snapshot of what healthcare clients (hospitals, physicians, public health officials) believe are their top priorities.

F I G U R E   1-3

Health Information Technology Priorities in 2003, 2004, and 2006

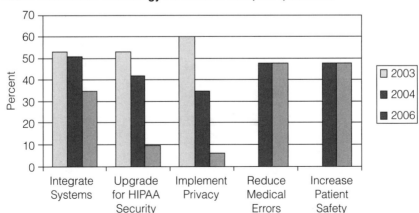

HIPAA indicates Health Insurance Portability and Accountability Act of 1996.

Source: 15th Annual HIMSS Leadership Survey[41] sponsored by Superior Consultant Company.

FIGURE 1-4

Health Information Technology Priorities in 2006

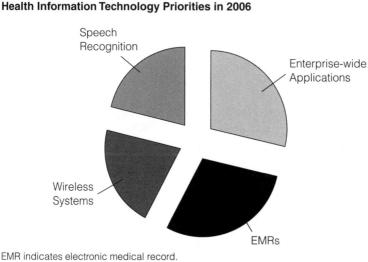

EMR indicates electronic medical record.

Source: 15th Annual HIMSS Leadership Survey[41] sponsored by Superior Consultant Company.

START EMR IMPLEMENTATION WITH A PLAN

Getting started is the hard part. Once the move to electronic medical records is underway, everyone will follow a well-defined plan.

FIGURE 1-5

Business Issues in 2003 and 2006

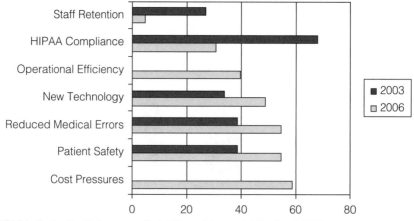

HIPAA indicates Health Insurance Portability and Accountability Act of 1996.

Source: 15th Annual HIMSS Leadership Survey[41] sponsored by Superior Consultant Company.

Step 1: Appoint an Electronic Health Record Physician Advocate

Every physician's office, regardless of size, needs one physician to see EHR/EMR implementation through completion. The EHR advocate must embrace not only a technology change but a culture change as well. Mark Anderson, founder of the AC Group and healthcare IT futurist, said, "If change is not embraced [from the practice leader], the probability of success is very low."

Step 2: Establish an Electronic Medical Records Implementation Team

In a large practice, the implementation team may be several physicians and the health information management team. In a smaller practice, it includes the HIPAA security official, a technology-competent physician, medical and billing records workforce member, and an independent IT consultant with no financial ties to an EMR vendor. A physician who champions the move to EMRs must lead the team. A critical factor in successful EMR implementation is to have at least one physician take the lead for the office. EMR implementation cannot be delegated to the office staff because it also involves how the physician makes clinical decisions.

Step 3: Determine an Adoption Plan and Timeline

In determining your adoption plan and timeline, include a plan to conduct parallel electronic and paper medical records. (You'll find more details on timelines and paperless plans in Chapters 2 and 3.) Do you intend to go paperless in six months, two years, or all at once? Consult your practice's privacy and security officials to ensure that your HIPAA privacy and security policies and procedure are in place early in your timeline and that your privacy and security officials have a plan to safeguard protected health information during the transition from paper to electronic format.

Step 4: Establish a Want List

Your want list should be specific to your practice and specialty. Prioritize items on the list. This list is likely to change as you progress through the EMR search, but establish a starting point. Even though practices and their workflows differ, EMRs have been around long enough in a variety of practices to establish commonalities among practices, making it easier for EMR vendors to accommodate your want list.

Step 5: Evaluate Your Onsite and Offsite Business Partners That Send and Receive Electronic Health Records

What outside resources do you depend upon to stay in business? Your business partners may include coders, billing services, labs, hospitals, pharmacies, clearinghouses, or other physician offices. More important, from cost and return-on-investment perspectives, which of these resources do you need and which could the EHR replace? For example, by going to an electronic format, most practices can eliminate outside transcription fees.

Step 6: Review Research Reports and Electronic Medical Record Studies

Each year, several organizations evaluate EMR applications to assist physicians in making decisions about what to purchase. Two reports in particular are worth reviewing:

- The *Information Technology Trends and Solutions: Extensive Evaluation Ranks Top Electronic Health Records Applications* survey. A copy of this survey is included in Appendix C of this book and also can be found online at www.acgroup.org. The EMR trends study, conducted by the AC Group (www.acgroup.org), evaluated approximately 50 vendors based on 27 categories and four methods of operation. You'll notice in the Summary Results that a weighted point value was assigned to vendors with complete software applications. Often, when new technology emerges, several companies contribute technical capabilities to make a seamless product for the physician. Companies that blend technology tended not to rank as high as those with one single application. The study identified the top winners in the following categories:
  - A network of more than 100 physicians
  - Midsize practices with 15 to 99 physicians
  - Small practices with five to 15 physicians
  - Small practices with one to four physicians

- The *Annual Medical Records Institute Survey of Electronic Health Record Trends and Usage* provides the industry with "a balanced and objective measure of current EHR implementations and meaningful insights into market directions."[42] Researchers gathered responses from "all types of healthcare providers including those in ambulatory and acute care settings, Integrated Delivery Networks, Managed Care Organizations and other settings." (A summary report of findings is available at no cost at www.medrecinst.com.)

In addition, Physicians EHR, LLC (www.physiciansehr.com), provides a database of EMR software vendors and contact information for approximately 300 EMR vendors. The site also provides a "Demo Depot" for providers to preview several EHR demonstrations from one location. Physicians and practice managers can rate their experiences with EMR vendors and comment on several categories. You can review a vendor, add comments, or find vendor contacts at www. physiciansehr.com. Categories for physicians or practice managers to evaluate include:

- Ease of use and implementation
- Appropriate for practice size
- Cost compatible with budget
- Met, or is meeting, return-on-investment promises
- Training and technical assistance provided by vendor including:
    - Cost
    - Knowledge and customer support
    - Availability when needed
- Interoperability with other specialties, labs, hospitals

Step 7: Evaluate Your Current Technology Capabilities

Are your computers more than four years old? If so, a comprehensive EHR software package could lock up your system or your system may lack necessary security to protect electronic protected health information. Hardware is often the least expensive investment in an EHR, but it can create the biggest headaches if it isn't current and regularly maintained and updated, as appropriate.

What kind of hardware is on your want list? This could include personal computers for office and exam rooms, a central database server, network hardware, and modems. Does the practice want to use wireless technology? What devices does the clinical staff want to work with (eg, tablets, personal computers, personal data assistants [PDAs], laptops)? Some decisions regarding hardware are driven by the EMR application and vendor that your practice selects.

How many computers will need Internet access? If you use wireless technology, where should you place your antennae? What security issues should your security official address prior to making a selection? (Chapter 3 offers more details about assessing technology capabilities.)

Step 8: Forecast Your Budget

It may be premature to determine a budget if you are just starting your EMR research. However, preliminary estimates can help you begin planning. You can then adjust those estimates to reflect your practice's identified needs.

The cost to purchase hardware, modems, preinstallation planning and implementation training, software support (usually an annual contract), software licenses (usually one per physician), hardware and network support ranges from $15,000 to $50,000 per physician, according to the AC Group.[43]

We've seen innovative business models that help physicians share EMR costs with a community of healthcare providers. Web-based models may charge $99 to $700 per month per physician in addition to a user fee. Monthly fees can be difficult to estimate if the fee is dependent upon use. (We discuss budgeting and purchasing decision in Chapter 3.)

SUMMARY

Poll findings on physician adoption of EMRs vary widely, ranging from 3% to 24% of the physician population already in the implementation stage. An important key to success of EMR implementation in your practice is that it's in your budget for the next two years and that you interview several vendors before making a final EMR selection decision.

In Chapter 2, we take a look at administrative and clinical workflows that are triggered by paper in a paper-based environment. Then, we show you screenshots from several vendors so you can see how workflows look in an EMR setting.

In Chapter 3, we provide guidance on making the EMR purchase, identify business purchase models that are friendly to the physician's budget, look at a sample request for proposal (RFP), and discuss on what you should expect as a return on investment.

In closing, we offer the words of John Haughom, MD, at the HIMSS Conference in Orlando in early 2004, as reported in *Healthcare Informatics*:

> The determinants of success for implementing an EMR boil down to four things:
>
> ■ Vision and leadership
> ■ People
> ■ Process
> ■ Partnerships
>
> Putting in the EMR for us was a necessary step to deal with the quality and safety issues that exist in healthcare.[14]

ENDNOTES

1. Remarks of Senator Hillary Rodham Clinton on the *Health Information for Quality Improvement Act*, January 12, 2004. Available at: http://clinton.senate.gov/~clinton/speeches/2004112651.html.

2. Definition provided by the American Academy of Family Physicians (www.aafp.org).

3. Definition provided by the Healthcare Information and Management Systems Society (www.himss.org).

4. Definition provided by the Delaware Healthcare Association Glossary of Healthcare Terms and Acronyms (www.deha.org/Glossary/GlossaryB.htm).

5. Definition provided by *Webster's Online Dictionary* (www.webster-dictionary.org).

6. Definition provided by the e-Health Initiative through the National Health Information Infrastructure (www.nhii.org).

7. Adams K, Corrigan JM, eds. *Priority Areas for National Action: Transforming Healthcare Quality.* Washington, DC: National Academy Press; 2003.

8. Institute of Medicine. *Crossing the Quality Chasm: A New Health System for the 21st Century.* Washington, DC: National Academy Press; 2001.

9. Institute of Medicine. Crossing the quality chasm: the IOM Health Care Quality Initiative. Available at: www.iom.edu/focuson.asp?id=8089.

10. The Institute of Medicine. The IOM Quality Initiative: a progress report at year six. *Shaping the Future: Newsletter of the IOM.* 2002;1. Available at: www.iom.edu/Object.File/Master/7/612/0.pdf.

11. "Level Seven" refers to the highest level of the International Standards Organization's (ISO) communications model for open systems interconnection (OSI)—the application level. For more information about HL7 standards go to www.HL7.org.

12. For more information about the EHR Collaborative go to www.ehrcollaborative.org.

13. "EMRs for Small Physician Groups," a report by Forrester Research, Inc, December 2003. For more information go to www.forrester.com.

14. Hagland M. Reality EMRs: coming soon to an organization near you—electronic record keeping. *Healthcare Informatics.* 2004;21:36.

15. Conn J. Health IT czar mulls financial options. *Modern Phys.* 2004;6.

16. Secretary Thompson, seeking fastest possible results, names first health information technology coordinator [news release]. Washington, DC: US Department of Health and Human Services; May 6, 2004. Available at: www.hhs.gov/news/press/2004pres/20040506.html.

17. Brailer DJ, Terasawa E. "Use and Adoption of Computer-based Patient Records," report prepared for the California Healthcare Foundation, October 2003.

18. Thompson TG, Brailer DJ. The decade of health information technology: delivering consumer-centric and information-rich care, framework for strategic action. Available at: www.hhs.gov/onchit/framework.

19. Physician's electronic health record coalition (PEHRC) [news release]. Washington, DC: Center for Health Information Technology; August 19, 2004. Available at: www.centerforhit.org/x199.xml.

20. David J. Brailer, MD, PhD, in discussion with author (CPH), August 13, 2004.

21. Austin M. Process eases patient's access to medical records. *Denver Post.* June 25, 2004.

22. Hagland M. Reality EMRs: coming soon to an organization near you—electronic record keeping. *Healthcare Informatics.* 2004;21:36.

23. For more information about HIPAA's Privacy and Security Rules, consult *HIPAA Plain & Simple: A Compliance Guide for Healthcare Professionals* by Carolyn P. Hartley and Edward D. Jones III (AMA Press, 2004).

24. This is just one example of interoperability. Of course, information on the EHR could be transmitted in a secure fashion over the Internet or with authorized access by the referred physician visiting the referring physician's Web site and accessing the record directly.

25. "2004 Survey of Physicians 50 to 65 Years Old, Based on 2003 Data," a summary report by Merritt, Hawkins & Associates. Available at: www.merritthawkins.com/compensation_surveys.cfm.

26. To go on a visual tour of Central Utah's Multi-Specialty Clinic, go to www.touchworksemr.com/_htm/TW_CaseStudies.asp.

27. Kranhold K. Group of companies to expand information technology bonus program for physicians. *Wall Street Journal.* May 26, 2004.

28. Medicare Announces Initiatives to Improve Care and Provide New Services Through Information Technology [news release]. Washington, DC: Centers for Medicare and Medicaid Services; July 17, 2004. Available at www.cms.hhs. gov/media/press/release.asp?Counter=1117.

29. CMS Studies Confirm Significant Savings Through Medicare-Approved Drug Discount Cards. Washington, DC: Centers for Medicare and Medicaid Services; October 12, 2004. Available at www.cms.hhs.gov/medicarereform/drugcard/reports/CMSDrugCardAnalysis.pdf.

30. William Davis, MD in discussion with the author (CPH).

31. Garcia, AM. Electronic medical records: content, community, and commerce [white paper]. Available at: www.drnotes.com/news_articles/EMRContentCommunityCommerce051004.pdf.

32. Doug Holmes, MD, in discussion with the author (CPH).

33. Landro L. The doctor is online: secure messaging boosts the use of web consultations. *Wall Street Journal.* September 2, 2004.

34. A new CPT code lets you get reimbursed for online patient evaluation. *Physician's e-Health Report.* May/June 2004.

35. California Healthcare Foundation. Program would allow physicians to monitor patients via cell phone. *iHealthBeat.* June 16, 2004. Available at: http://ihealthbeat.org.

36. Rand study shows people at risk of receiving poor healthcare in all parts of the United States [news release]. Washington, DC: RAND Corporation; May 4, 2004.

37. Barrett MJ, Holmes BJ, McAulay SE. "Electronic Medical Records: A Buyer's Guide for Small Physician Practices." A report prepared for California Healthcare Foundation by Forrester Research Inc, October 2003.

38. EMR vendors provide case studies on their Web sites for physician review. The communications department at SynaMed referred us to Inderpal Chabra's comments available at www.synamed.com.

39. What docs want in an EMR. *Physician's e-Health Report.* May/June 2004.

40. The "15th Annual Health Information and Management Systems Society Leadership Survey" can be found at www.himss.org.

41. Respondents to this survey were attendees and exhibitors at HIMSS' annual conferences and likely represent a more technologically inclined response than nonparticipants.

42. Medical Record Institute. Sixth Annual Medical Records Institute Survey of Electronic Health Record Trends and Usage. Available at: www.medrecinst. com/pages/latestNews.asp?id=99.

43. Anderson MR. Information technology trends and solutions [white paper]. May 27, 2004. (This report is available in the appendix of this book.)

chapter 2

An Electronic Medical Record System: Your Electronic Workflow Assistant in the Medical Office

Eighty-three percent of office administrators and financial advisors responding to a 2003 Medical Research Institute survey said the need to improve workflow was the number one motivating factor for implementing an electronic medical record (EMR) system.[1] However, when selecting an EMR system for your office, you should first determine whether the EMR is capable of handling administrative and clinical workflow management for a practice of your size and specialty and still allow for growth. It should allow you to review and process clinical documents, which are the keys to improved patient safety, improved decision making, and improved billing and coding. Long after the sales representative and training teams have left your office, your workflow partner will be your EMR software applications, and that partner needs to dependably show up for work whether you're in or out of the office.

In this chapter, we take a look at several administrative and clinical workflow modules so that you can see how the work flows in a paper-based environment and what that same workflow process looks like in an electronic environment. (Figure 2-1 illustrates the approach we take to each module.) We also illustrate, through computer screenshots, the various EMR applications available. With these screenshots you can see how the electronic process looks and how it can simplify the workflow of the paper-based office.

WHAT YOU WILL LEARN IN THIS CHAPTER

- What is workflow and why it is important
- How to parlay your administrative workflow into an EMR

■ How to parlay your clinical workflow into an EMR

■ How to involve patients in your EMR workflow

FIGURE 2-1

A Roadmap for This Chapter

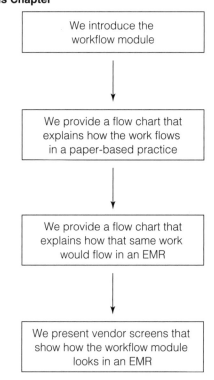

EMR indicates electronic medical record.

Key Terms[2]

Clinical Decision Support: Typically used when referring to a type of system that assists healthcare providers in making medical decisions. These types of systems typically require input of patient-specific clinical variables and as a result provide patient-specific recommendations.

Clinical Information: Refers to the data contained in the patient record. The data may include information such as problem lists, lab results, current medications, family history, patient identification, and insurance information.

Clinical Pathway: A standardized plan of care against which health performance and progress is measured. A clinical pathway shows exact timing of all key patient care activities intended to achieve expected standard outcomes within designated time frames. A clinical pathway includes documentation of problems, expected outcomes and goals, and clinical interventions and orders.

Encounter: A face-to-face meeting between an individual seeking healthcare treatment and a healthcare provider whose services are provided.

Workflow is what happens as a result of workforce members following an established path to reach a common outcome. In the medical office, there are two primary types of workflow: administrative and clinical. In the following steps, we evaluate how they are interdependent, and how to manage changes during the early stages of implementation.

STEP 1: EVALUATE YOUR WORKFLOW TO UNDERSTAND WHAT WILL CHANGE

If you ask a physician what the office manager does, the answer is likely to be, "I don't know, but I can't get along without her." If you ask an office manager what she does in a physician's office, the answer is likely to be, "Anything that needs to be done. I've been the receptionist, file clerk, medical records clerk, in-house sleuth searching for patient charts, staff psychologist, FMLA/EEOC/Privacy/Security officer, patient complaint department. . . ."

In a small to midsize physician office, responsibilities usually overlap among workforce members and everyone is likely to know how to step in when needed. "Other duties as assigned" is the rule rather than the exception.

In a practice that relies on paper, the presence of "paper" has been a visual indication that something needs to happen, from sticky notes on the front of a medical chart to a stack of charts on the physician's desk. But making the switch from a paper-based office to a nearly paperless office involves planning, preparation, training, and a physician "champion" to facilitate the changes in office culture, procedures, staffing assignments, and records management.

Here are some examples of these visual signs or "triggers."

In a practice that relies on an EMR, the visual cues are on the computer screen rather than posted on a wall or taking up space in a records room,

Example 1

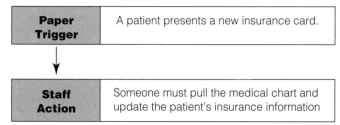

Example 2

Paper Trigger	A medical chart hangs in a slot on the exam door

↓

Staff Action	The nurse completed an initial exam and the patient is inside, waiting for the doctor

Example 3

Workforce Member: Paper-Based	**Workforce Member: Electronic Medical Record**		
I am the process (does the work)	I am the process tender (oversees movement of documents)		
If it happens, it's because I physically made it happen	Document Imaging	Chart Management	Order Entry

EMR indicates electronic medical record.

the practice's kitchen, or message center. Workforce members who once made the process happen in a paper world will become process tenders in an EMR environment and verify that the process has been done.

Let's examine an easy paper workflow example (Figure 2-2).[3] Here, a patient checks into a small family practice and, based on what the patient indicated on the phone, the receptionist scheduled the patient for a limited visit. Note that the paper triggers an administrative workload that advances the flow of information. For discussion purposes, let's say the workflow for a patient to arrive and meet with a doctor is this easy. Most medical practices don't give much thought to paper-based workflow because the practice has established its management and billing processes and cultural habits.

All too often, EMR consultants hear, "We do it like this because it works," or, "this is the way we've always done it." But even in a loose environment, someone made workflow decisions for a reason:

■ The doctor or office manager likes it that way
■ Regulations require it
■ Assigned tasks are compatible with workforce member's skills

You may ask, "If the system works, why fix it?" The problem is that reports such as those from the RAND study and the Institute of Medicine provide evidence that the paper system isn't working.

When changing from paper-based processes to an EMR, the practice has the opportunity to critically evaluate its workflows for an electronic

F I G U R E 2-2

Workflow: Patient Arrives to See the Doctor, Paper-Based Environment

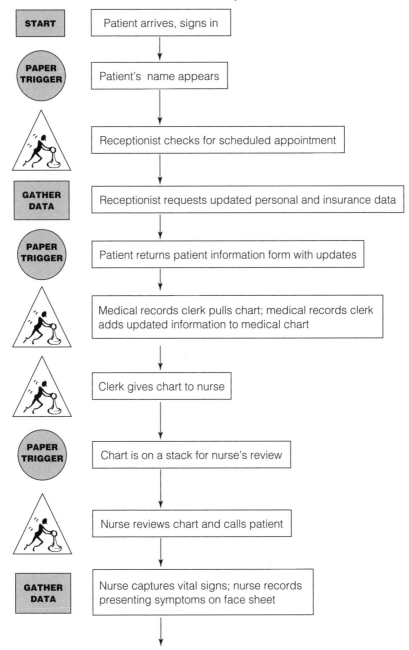

continued

F I G U R E   2-2

Workflow: Patient Arrives to See the Doctor, Paper-Based Environment cont'd

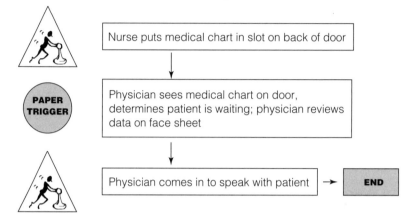

environment. Many administrative and operational workflows may be significantly simplified.

Although not all EMRs work the same way, the process to move a patient through the office is similar. The workflow in an EMR can be reduced to three or four action items. In Figure 2-3, notice that there are only four actions required of administrative and clinical staff. All other activity is managed by the EMR. Remember the EMR is the electronic filing cabinet and the electronic health record (EHR) is the interoperable electronic health record.

In the electronic workflow example shown in Figure 2-3, the practice staff physically handles two tasks:

- The receptionist greets the patient and verifies updated patient data.
- The nurse brings the patient into the exam room and gathers vitals and presenting symptoms.

STEP 2: MAP YOUR PAPER WORKFLOW

A practice that defines its workflow processes in a manner similar to that in Step 1 has a better chance of successfully transitioning into an electronic environment than a practice that "isn't sure how things happen, it just all works out."

The same activities that occur in a paper-based office also occur in an electronic practice; the only difference is that the EMR automatically and transparently conducts many of the activities. In Figure 2-3, the EMR completed the following administrative activities upon command:

- Logged the patient into the office
- Gathered and updated patient's personal demographic information

- Pulled the charts from the scheduler software and presented them to the nurse
- Updated the medical record with new clinical data
- Moved the charts along to the physician
- Incorporated the charts in the patient's medical record when the doctor was finished with the patient

Let's take another look at the check-in process when the patient is involved in the process. The touch screen used when the patient checks in

FIGURE 2-3

Workflow: Patient Arrives to See the Doctor, EMR

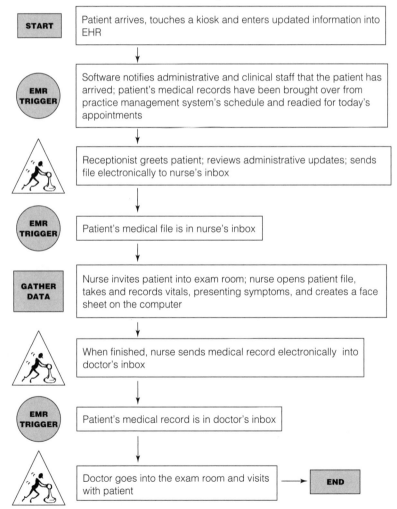

EHR indicates electronic health record; EMR, electronic medical record.

FIGURE   2-4

Patient Portal From A4 Health Systems. A patient provides online information before an office visit and completes a questionnaire.

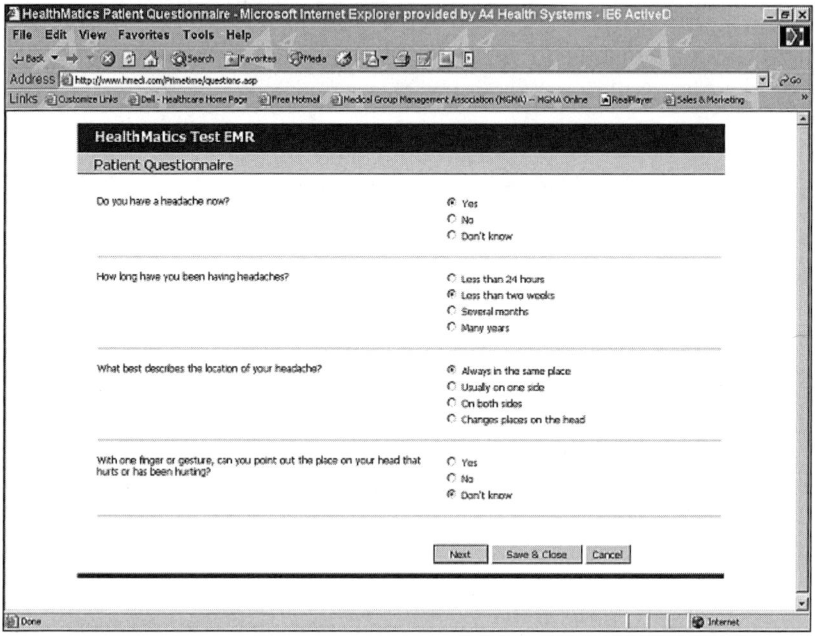

How to read this screen: (1) Patient logs in from the Web or the waiting room. (2) Patient gives reason for visit or completes the questionnaire. (3) After questionnaire is completed, the EMR is populated with patient data and feeds data to the front desk. (4) Physician begins visit with patient's subjective history already complete, nearly 10% of total documentation. (5) Physician reviews and confirms information.

Reprinted with permission from A4 Health Systems (www.a4healthsystems.com).[4]

may look like the one in Figure 2-4. Here, the patient enters pertinent medical history and the reason for the visit.

As you will see in this chapter, not all software systems look alike. Some physicians prefer the look and function of one screen over another. In the next example (Figures 2-5 and 2-6), the patient can also use a touch screen or enter data from another Web site.

Figure 2-7 illustrates a system that pulls together several administrative functions onto one "desktop." You can see that there are four people in separate exam rooms. Three wait to see the nurse, and one waits to see the doctor.[5]

Most software applications allow the practice administrator to do the following:

■ View workloads for each clinical and administrative workforce member

F I G U R E 2-5

Patient Portal (1) From SynaMed

Reprinted courtesy SynaMed (www.synamed.com).[6]

F I G U R E 2-6

Patient Portal (2) From SynaMed

Reprinted courtesy SynaMed (www.synamed.com).[6]

- Track patient movement
- Obtain a bird's-eye view of the information flow

With an EMR, the software can track information, but *software is no replacement for personal contact.* Even top-of-the-line software is no substitute for the interpersonal dynamics that keep practice members working together with patients as a unified team.

STEP 3: EVALUATE WORK MODULES FOR A LAYERED ADOPTION OF AN ELECTRONIC HEALTH RECORD SYSTEM

All EMR systems are not created equal. Some work better for large practice networks, others work well for specialties, and some are appropriate for solo and small physician practices. An EMR can be software based, while others are hosted on the Web. Some vendors call the process of building medical files "charting" and others call it "data entry."

The transition from paper-based to electronic format involves several layers of change management in financial, administrative, and cultural areas. A small group of practitioners will have fewer workforce members

FIGURE 2-7

Patients Wait in Exam Room. In this HealthMatics® EMR screen by A4 Health Systems, notice the visual cue that a patient is ready to see the doctor in the exam room. It looks like this: Manning, Te . . . Exam Room 4 Perget, Roy 4/19/2004 12:00 AM.

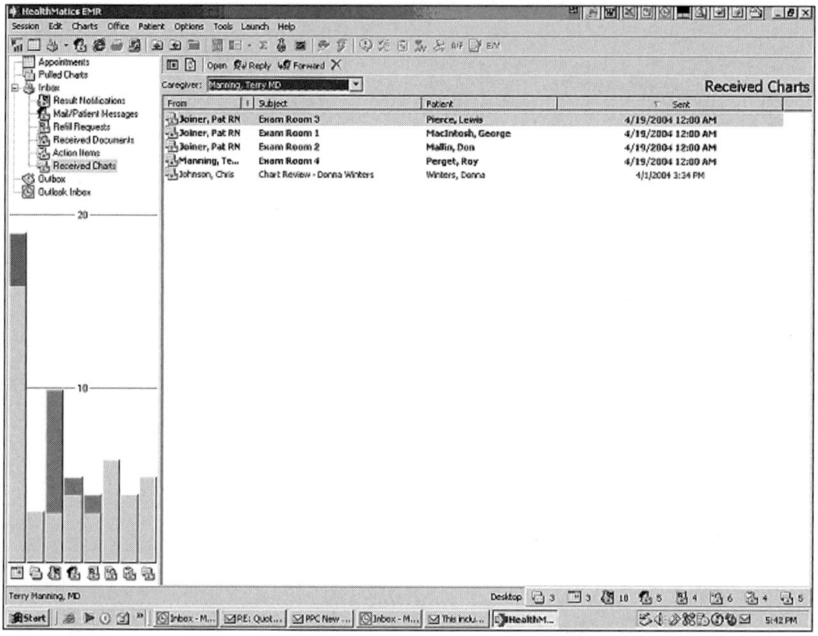

How to read this screen: (1) On the bottom left side of this screen, you see six bars with miniature icons below each bar. These icons are located just above Terry Manning, MD's name on the lower left screen. A4 Health Systems calls these bars "stacks," similar to paper files that "stack up" in a paper-based office. (2) The first stack represents the physician's schedule. According to this first bar, the physician will see 21 patients today, and the shaded area indicates the doctor has seen approximately 20% of today's patients. (3) The second stack includes the pooled chart stack. In a paper-based office, this would be the stacks of patient charts that a physician would carry under his or her arm or that workforce members would move around the office during the day. This bar contains compiled medical charts for patients on today's schedule. (4) Lab work and test results are the third stack. The shaded portion (in red on a color computer) appears to have about seven out of 10 lab results awaiting review as abnormal and needing attention. (5) The fourth stack contains messages within the practice that need a response. (6) The fifth stack is for prescriptions. Here, the physician can pull up the patient record, evaluate current prescriptions, and, using a password, fax a new prescription or refill to the patient's pharmacy. (7) The final stack represents action items. Here, physicians and workforce members can check the status of internal tasks that have been assigned. Reprinted with permission from A4 Health Systems (www.a4healthsystems.com).[4]

to engage in the transition than a multispecialty, multilocation network, but each will experience similar challenges in the transition process.

Some practices choose to purchase an EMR software license and integrate the software with existing systems. Other practices prefer to pay a monthly user's fee. In both cases, EMRs are best adopted in modules, and both decisions are driven primarily by budget and need.

Workflow Module: Scheduler

Let's begin as you would usually start the day, by taking a look at the patient load and office schedule. In the screen shown in Figure 2-8, Mary Jones, MD, is checking in to view her day's lineup of patients by appointment time.[7] With this application on the Web, Dr Jones can view her schedule from a wireless computer, the office's networked computers, the hospital, or her home.

FIGURE 2-8

eClinicalWorks Provided Online by IntegriMED Shows the Status of Today's Office Visits

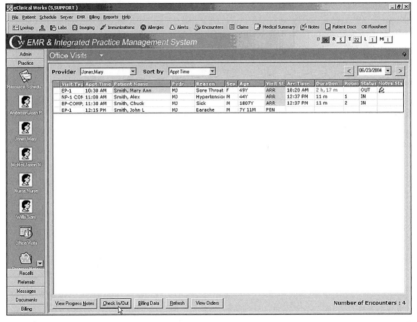

How to read this screen: (1) When Dr Mary Jones checks into this screen, she can preview patients scheduled for the day, first by visit type and appointment time. (2) Highlighted portions on this screen show her that "Mary Ann Smith" has already been seen and has left the office. (3) Alex Smith's and Chuck Smith's Visit Status, ARR, is highlighted to let the doctor know that they have arrived (ARR). A quick glance at the Visit Type (far left) lets Dr Jones know how best to prepare for each of the patient visits. (4) The Duration column lets Dr Jones know how long the patient has been waiting, and the Room column tells her where to find each patient. (5) Dr Jones double-clicks on the patient name to obtain presenting concerns for today's visit, and she also checks for allergies, immunizations, and alerts.

Reprinted with permission from eClinicalWorks, available online through IntegriMED[SM] (www.integrimed.com).[8]

Notice that patient Alex Smith is in Waiting Room 1. The stethoscope icon at the end of the screen indicates that the nurse has completed taking the vitals and that the patient is ready to be seen by the physician. This electronic workflow indicator replaces the paper chart placed in the slot on the door or the colored flags outside the exam room.

Workflow Module: e-Prescribing Management

E-Prescribing has been around for more than two decades, but since 2003, e-prescribing adoption has grown from "nice to have" to "got to have." The Health Insurance Portability and Accountability Act of 1996 (HIPAA) Privacy and Security Rules, along with community-wide disease management studies, homeland security issues, and public health concerns, are driving e-prescribing technology to be continually refined. Further, the Medicare Modernization Act, signed by President Bush in December 2003, provides for a federally standardized system of e-prescribing to be in place nationwide by the end of this decade.

The face of e-prescribing in the physician's office is as much a safety issue as it is a workflow issue. Certainly physicians in general have developed a less-than-favorable reputation for penmanship. While many print by hand or use prestamped prescriptions, the prescription remains on paper and is only recorded into the patient's medical chart when someone takes the time to write it in. And just because a prescription is added to the paper chart doesn't mean the medication record will be easily seen each time a physician flips through the chart looking for drug interactions, adverse reactions, or duplicate renewals.

The actions required to renew or refill a prescription involve both administrative and clinical workflow. All too often the prescription renew process becomes a huge headache. In a paper-based office, the renew prescription workflow looks something like the flowchart shown in Figure 2-9.

Administrative workflow in this relatively simple renewal request involved 10 steps, and each step required a nurse, medical records workforce member, and a physician to take action, all the while keeping track of where the patient's record was last seen. Meanwhile, the patient has gone to the pharmacy only to learn that the prescription has not yet been *called* in. The result is usually an irritated patient or pharmacist calling the doctor's office.

Before calling in the prescription, the nurse or physician usually searches for medical files at another nurse's station or under a pile of medical charts. Or worse, the physician writes a sticky note indicating a renewal needs to be ordered. What happens next? The note falls off the file and the renewal never gets documented or, worse, the prescription is called in for another patient.

F I G U R E   2-9

Workflow to Renew a Prescription: Paper-Based Practice

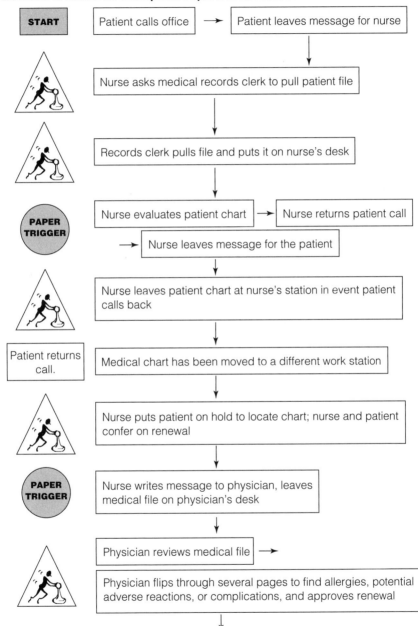

continued

FIGURE 2-9

Workflow to Renew a Prescription: Paper-Based Practice cont'd.

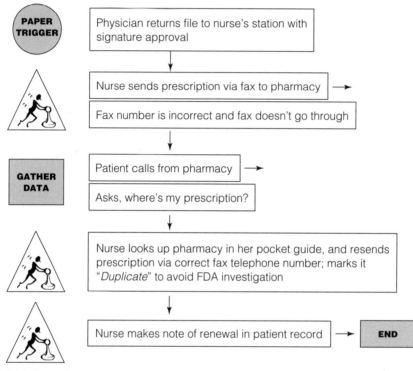

FDA indicates Food and Drug Administration.

One of the most attractive features of an EHR is e-prescribing, including writing, tracking and renewing prescriptions. The EHR combines the safety of e-prescribing with reduced administrative workflow. That's why the task of monitoring prescriptions is usually at the top of the physician's EMR request list.

In an EMR workflow model, we can see how data are stored without getting lost or misplaced. The process improves clinical documentation, patient satisfaction, and patient safety. The process to renew a prescription using an EMR should look like the process outlined in Figure 2-10.

The brevity of this shortened administrative and clinical workflow is enough to delight any nurse who has been the communications traffic cop between patient and physician on prescription renewals. In the following set of screenshots, we show you what this prescription renewal transaction looks like on the computer screen, starting with Figure 2-11, which illustrates how a telephone encounter is handled.

FIGURE 2-10

Workflow to Refill a Prescription: EMR

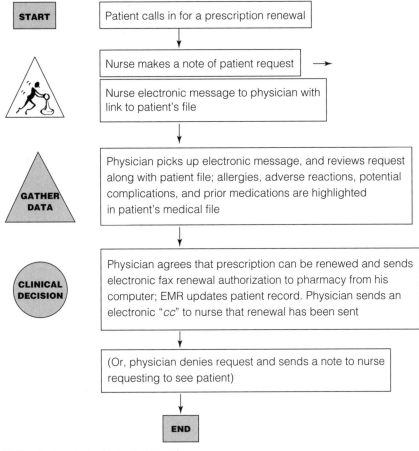

EMR indicates electronic medical record.

In Figure 2-12, you see in the background that Dr Willis has opened Alex Smith's medical record.

Some physicians prefer to use handheld devices when reviewing medical charts or e-prescribing. Figure 2-13 shows the physician prescribing 125 mg of chewable amoxicillin to a 29-year-old patient with acute bronchitis.

In Figure 2-14, the physician uses a laptop to fill or renew a prescription. On a color screen, you see the smiley face, frown face, and straight-mouthed face, which indicate the status of the patient's prescription insurance program.

FIGURE 2-11

EMR Telephone Encounter, Prescription Refill, Part 1

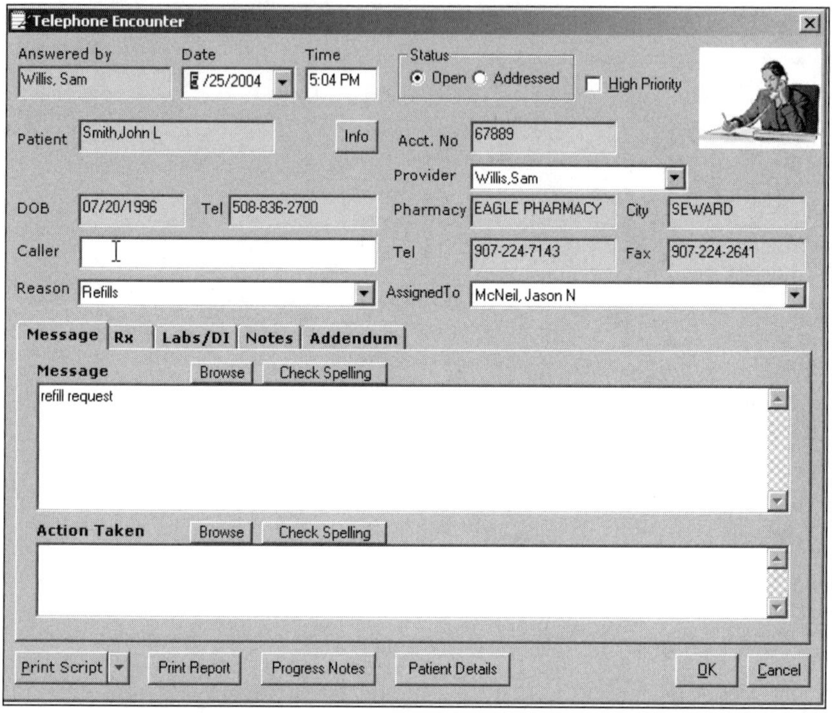

How to read this screen: In this telephone encounter, the nurse sends a message to Dr Sam Willis about patient Alex Smith. In the middle of this screen, you can see that Alex Smith's pharmacy information (city, telephone number, and fax number) was added to the system during an earlier visit.

Reprinted with permission from eClinicalWorks offered online by IntegriMED (www.intregrimed.com).[8]

FIGURE 2-12

EMR Telephone Encounter, Prescription Refill, Part 2

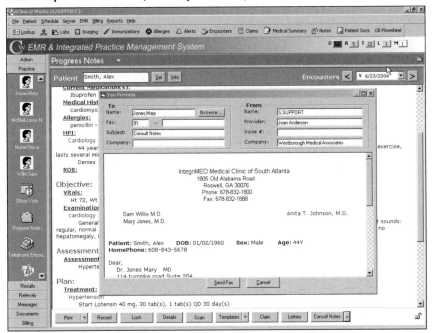

How to read this screen: The screen in the foreground shows that Dr Willis has approved the prescription refill for patient Alex Smith and is preparing to send an electronic fax to the pharmacy. At the same time, Dr Willis will send a copy of the refill order to his physician partner, Mary Jones, MD.

Reprinted with permission from eClinicalWorks, offered online by IntegriMED (www.integrimed.com).[8]

FIGURE 2-13

Prescription Renewal on a Handheld Computing Device Using TouchWorks From Allscripts Healthcare Solutions

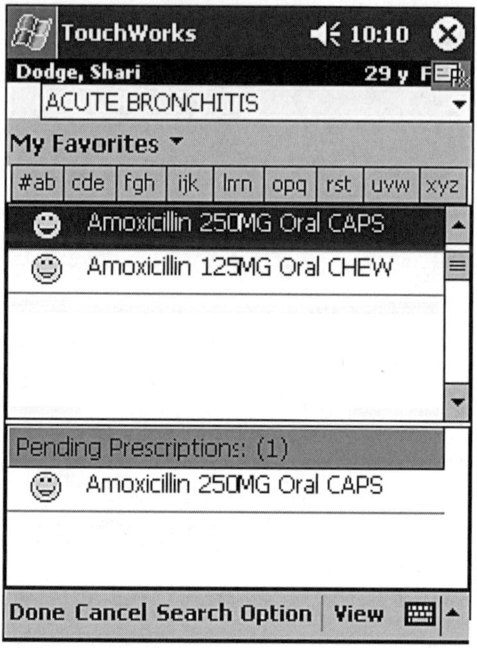

How to read this handheld screen: (1) The physician can renew an existing prescription or write a new prescription by reviewing a medication list catalogued either by diagnosis or a preferred list in alphabetical order. (2) Here, the physician selected "My Favorites" and then selected two dosages of "Amoxicillin" filed under the #ab tab. For this particular patient, the doctor selects 125MG instead of 250MG. (3) To the left of Amoxicillin, you see a smiley face. On the full-color handheld screen, you'll see a green face that indicates this prescription will be accepted by the patient's insurance formulary. (4) A red frown indicates that the prescription is not accepted by the patient's insurance. The physician can explain to the patient why it is the drug of choice and prescribe it anyway or select another prescription. (5) A yellow straight-mouthed face indicates the payer will cover the prescription, but it comes with a higher copayment. (6) Similar to other EHRs, TouchWorks warns the physician not to prescribe medication when the patient has experienced an allergic or adverse reaction.

Reprinted with permission from Allscripts Healthcare Solutions (www.allscripts.com).[9]

FIGURE 2-14

Prescription Renewal From a Browser on a Desktop or Mobile Laptop Computer Using TouchWorks From Allscripts Healthcare Solutions

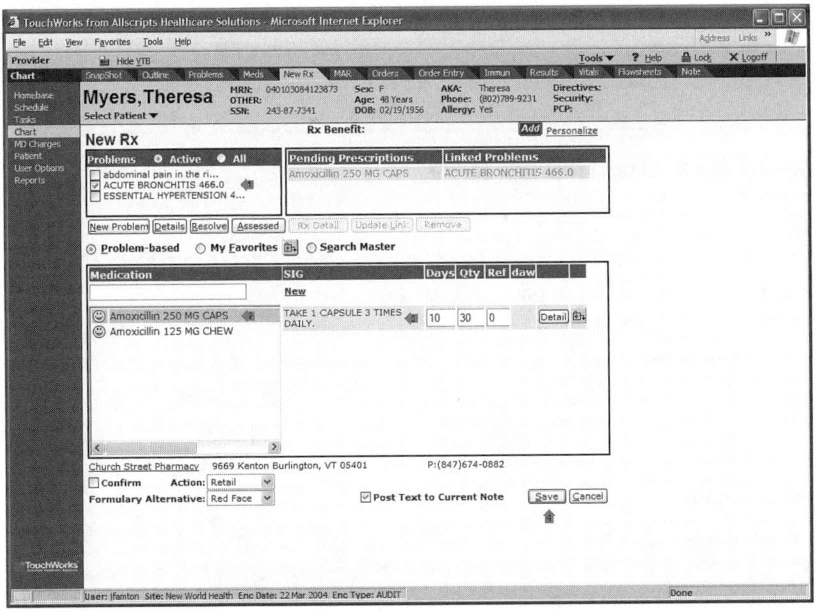

How to read this screen: This screen shows the same pharmacy renewal transaction on a desktop or laptop that also appear on the handheld device. (1) Notice you can click across the top of the screen to provide the physician with a snapshot of the patient's medical chart. The section that is opened is the prescription or "Rx" tab. (2) Arrows (red on a color screen) highlight three areas to check before refilling the prescription: the diagnosis, the selected dosage of amoxicillin (notice the smiley face indicates whether the prescription is on the insured's formulary), and instructions on how often to take this prescription.

Reprinted with permission from Allscripts Healthcare Solutions (www.allscripts.com).[9]

Taking the Pain Out of a Pharmaceutical Recall

One sure way to disrupt workflow comes when a manufacturer recalls a drug. On September 30, 2004, Merck & Co, Inc recalled its arthritis and acute pain drug, VIOXX®, an event that affected approximately 20 million United States patients.

North Fulton Family Medicine, a 16-provider, multisite family practice in Alpharetta, Georgia, serves more than 330 patients per day. Its staff faced the enormous task of notifying patients who had been prescribed VIOXX. To quickly identify all active patients on the medication, North Fulton Family Medicine utilized its EMR system's reporting module and queried the system using specific search criteria: "All active patients" + "VIOXX" + "All doses." The query electronically generated an 89-page report detailing all active patients taking the recalled drug, along with the patients' phone numbers.

continued

To convert patients to an alternative medication, the practice called each of the patients and scheduled a consultation. During each consultation, physicians relied on existing data in the medical record and cross-checked it against its Medispan® drug database for drug-drug and drug-allergy adverse reactions to alternative medication.

Medicare Comes of Age
By Ed Jones

Medicare Prescription Drug Improvement and Modernization Act of 2003 (MMA) is a whole lot more than a prescription drug program for seniors.

MMA (or DIMA) is the most comprehensive revision of the Medicare program since its inception almost 40 years ago. The table of contents alone is six pages long. The Medicare Prescription Drug Benefit is Title I. But you'll also find revisions to Medicare Advantage, Title II (formerly Medicare + Choice), Combating Fraud and Abuse (Title III), Provisions to Rural Provisions (Title IV), and on through a total of twelve titles.[10]

Three provisions are immediately capturing physicians' attention: physician fee schedule update, impact of expansion of Medicare coverage to pharmaceuticals, and electronic prescriptions.

Physician Fee Schedule
The Centers for Medicare and Medicaid Services (CMS) will increase payments to more than 875,000 physicians and other healthcare professionals for services under the Medicare Physician Fee Schedule by an average of more than 1.5% for calendar year 2004. These new revenue enhancing opportunities, effective January 1, 2004, are outlined in the January 7, 2004 *Federal Register*,[11] and they replace the November 2003 payment rates that would have reduced payment rates by an average of 4.5%.

Physicians in some rural and other areas will see an additional increase in payments, as Medicare payments in some areas of the country will rise by as much as 4.8%. A separate provision, affecting physicians in Alaska, will result in more than a 52% increase in average physician fee schedule payments for 2004.

Of particular note in MMA is *Section 413: Medicare Incentive Payment Program Improvements for Physician Scarcity*, which provides for a 5% bonus payment for physician services in designated rural areas from January 1, 2005 to December 31, 2007, furnished (a) by a primary care physician in a primary care scarcity county . . . ; or (b) by a physician who is not a primary care physician in a specialist care scarcity county.

To calculate your increase, go to www.cms.hhs.gov and select "Professionals." From the "Professionals" menu, select "Physicians." At this site, you'll find the Physicians Information Resource for Medicare, one of our "Editor's picks" because of its organization and understandability. Select "Physician's Fee Schedule" from the list and calculate your increase from one of the spread sheets at this site.

Prescription Drug Coverage

For the first time since inception of the Medicare program, prescription drug coverage (Medicare Part D) is offered to seniors under a *corridor of risk* premium plan, which goes into effect on January 1, 2006.

Medicare Part D provides Medicare beneficiaries with additional spending capabilities for a variety of pharmaceuticals. For some beneficiaries, the availability of Medicare Part D will free up disposable income that otherwise would be spent on healthcare maintenance. For others, who today might not be able to afford certain pharmaceuticals or related treatments, Medicare Part D opens new possibilities. For either group, Medicare Part D may increase demand for pharmaceutical related treatments, and hence, the demand for visits to physicians, such as initial preventive physical examinations (MMA, Section 611), cardiovascular screening blood tests (MMA, Section 612), diabetes screening tests (MMA, Section 613), and improved payment for certain mammography services (MMA, Section 614).

Another MMA provision permits home administration of some pharmaceuticals. In his article in the *Wall Street Journal*, Scott Hensley writes, "There are some high-priced drugs already covered because of quirks in how Medicare currently is administered. These include some medicines that must be given by a doctor in an office, including many cancer drugs. Under the new Medicare provision, drugs that can be taken orally or injected by patients at home also would be covered."[12]

MMA's pharmaceutical provisions have created high interest in the media since the White House announced an increase in cost from $400 billion to $534 billion over a ten-year period.

In 1965, the framers of Medicare predicted costs to run the nation's largest health-care system in 2000 would reach $10 billion. Early predictions weren't even close. Figures for 2000 came in at $240 billion.[13] So, it's no wonder financial forecasters fret over stability of the $534 billion price tag ten years from now.

Electronic Prescription Drug Program

Beginning in fiscal year 2007, which starts October 1, 2006, MMA authorizes the Secretary of the Department of Health and Human Services (HHS) to make grants to physicians to help them implement electronic prescription drug programs.[14]

An electronic prescription drug program, defined in *Section 101 (a): Medicare Prescription Drug Benefit*, is an important component of federal clinical initiatives, especially Secretary Thompson's endorsement of the electronic healthcare record in July 2003.[15] Electronic prescriptions also have the potential of enhancing patient safety and lowering administrative costs of physicians in maintaining and tracking pharmaceutical records for patients.

Under the MMA provisions, the Secretary of HHS "shall provide . . . for the promulgation of uniform standards relating to the requirements for electronic prescription drug programs. . . . Such standards shall be consistent with the objectives of improving

continued

(i) patient safety; (ii) the quality of care provided to patients; and (iii) efficiencies, including cost savings, in the delivery of care."[16]

Not later than September 1, 2005, the Secretary "shall develop, adopt, recognize, or modify initial uniform standards," taking into consideration any recommendations from the National Committee on Vital and Health Statistics (NCVHS), which in turn will reflect on any recommendations that have been provided from various stakeholders in the healthcare industry. Then, during a one-year period commencing January 1, 2006, the standards will be pilot tested by physicians and pharmacies that volunteer for the pilot. Following an evaluation of the pilot test results, the Secretary of HHS shall provide Congress a report on the evaluation by April 1, 2007, and promulgate by regulation final uniform electronic prescription drug standards by April 1, 2008.[14]

By the end of 2010, the healthcare industry will have uniform standards for electronic prescriptions. A number of states are considering state laws pertaining to electronic prescriptions now, but MMA provides that the final uniform federal standards take the place of "any State law or regulation that is contrary to the standards" or otherwise restrictive.[17]

Article reprinted with permission from the March/April 2004 issue of Physician's e-Health Report.[18]

Workflow Module: Billing and Coding

Approximately 90% of physicians responding to an early version of the 2004 American Academy of Family Physicians (AAFP) survey say they use a computer in the office, primarily to e-mail colleagues and access medical information on the Internet for patients.[19] But a computer alone with information about patients does not constitute an EMR. To meet your billing and coding module needs, the EMR you select must either:

- Integrate with your existing practice management system, or
- Add a robust billing and coding process to other modules.

A robust billing and coding system should include not only *International Classification of Diseases* (Ninth revision) (ICD-9) and Current Procedural Terminology (CPT®) codes, but also Systematized Nomenclature of Medicine and Current Terminology (SNOMED-CT), Healthcare Common Procedure Coding System (HCPCS), and Logical Observation Identifiers Names and Codes (LOINC). (These codes are discussed in Chapter 5.) Be sure to ask your practice management and EMR vendors how their systems will accommodate prospective migration to ICD-10 codes and new clinical standards such as SNOMED-CT and LOINC, if these codes are not already used in their systems.

Case Study: Overnight Adoption of EHRs

Jerry Bernstein, MD

Raleigh Pediatrics

When Jerry Bernstein, MD, pediatrician and EMR champion at Raleigh Pediatrics in North Carolina, was in the technology evaluation stage, he began looking for a system that would first bring efficiency to administrative workflow. Like most physicians, he was frustrated with sticky notes and misplaced medical files but primarily he was frustrated with payers who did not meet contractual obligations, thereby resulting in delayed payments and too many rejected claims.

He searched for a robust collections package that would:

- Keep payers on track with their negotiated contracts
- Assist in developing evaluation and management summaries
- Assign billing codes that significantly minimized rejected claims

After fighting for fair reimbursements for so many years, he was pleased with what he found.

Now, each of the 13 pediatricians at Raleigh Pediatrics carries a small laptop into each exam room and downloads patient records stored on the secure in-house server. After each patient visit, Dr Bernstein builds the evaluation and management summaries from templates, customizes those templates, and reviews the appropriate billing codes from the coding dictionaries.

Raleigh Pediatrics accepts insurance from six major payers. The practice maintains a staff of six billing and coding specialists; each specialist is assigned to one payer. "The software keeps us on the mark with ICD-9 and CPT codes, and each of the specialists maintains a relationship with one payer. That way, we've expedited reimbursements faster and more accurately," Dr Bernstein said. "When (not if, but when) there's a problem with a payer, we get billing colleagues who already know each other on the phone to solve the problem. Our argument is strengthened because we've got accessible data at our fingertips."

Figures 2-15, 2-16, and 2-17 display how a vendor helps physicians capture billing and coding information at the point of service. A robust collections module should recommend appropriate billing codes that are compatible with diagnostic codes. A companion module should evaluate the status of unpaid claims.

The next three screen shots (Figures 2-18, 2-19, and 2-20) show vendor samples of how a physician is able to capture charges at the point of service, analyze diagnostic and procedure codes, and recommend follow-up visits. The system automatically sends a reminder to either the scheduler or patient via e-mail.

FIGURE 2-15

Charge Capture at the Point of Service

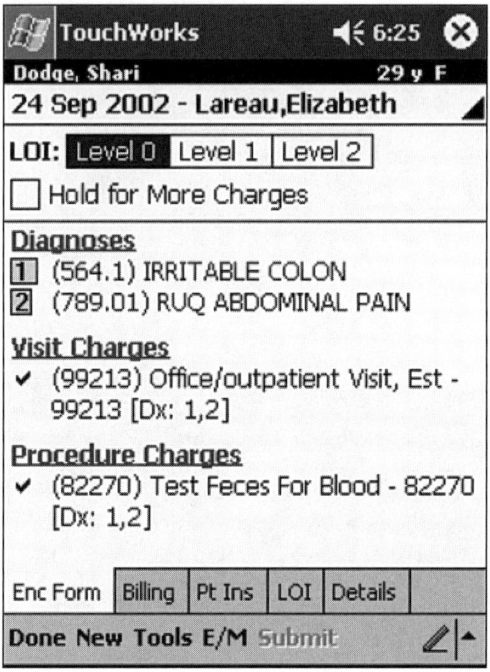

```
┌─────────────────────────────────────┐
│ 🎨 TouchWorks        🔊 6:25    ⊗   │
├─────────────────────────────────────┤
│ Dodge, Shari                 29 y F  │
│ 24 Sep 2002 - Lareau,Elizabeth    ◢ │
│ LOI: [Level 0] [Level 1] [Level 2]  │
│ ☐ Hold for More Charges              │
├─────────────────────────────────────┤
│ Diagnoses                            │
│ [1] (564.1) IRRITABLE COLON          │
│ [2] (789.01) RUQ ABDOMINAL PAIN      │
│                                      │
│ Visit Charges                        │
│ ✔ (99213) Office/outpatient Visit,   │
│   Est - 99213 [Dx: 1,2]              │
│                                      │
│ Procedure Charges                    │
│ ✔ (82270) Test Feces For Blood -     │
│   82270 [Dx: 1,2]                    │
├─────────────────────────────────────┤
│ Enc Form │ Billing │ Pt Ins │ LOI │ Details │
├─────────────────────────────────────┤
│ Done New Tools E/M Submit       ✎ ▴ │
└─────────────────────────────────────┘
```

How to read this screen: Here, the physician is capturing charges and building content to be added to the electronic patient chart. Physicians select a patient from their up-to-date personal schedule or patient rounding list. The software guides the physician through the selection of a diagnosis, visit, and procedural charge(s). Physicians simply review the charges and electronically submit them to the billing system. Depending on the level selected by the physician, the diagnostic and procedure codes will be adjusted and available for physician review and approval.

Reprinted with permission from Allscripts Healthcare Solutions (www.allscripts.com).[9]

FIGURE 2-16

Dictation on Handheld

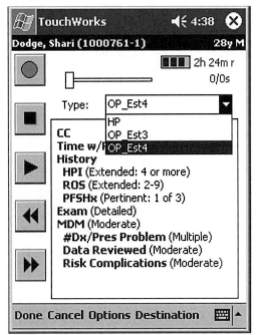

How to read this screen: This handheld is also a recorder. Here, the personal digital assistant (PDA) provides the physician the ability to record notes taken during the exam. Patient demographic and appointment information is tied to the digital recording and can be displayed at the tap of a button, while guiding physicians through the dictation process with custom-built dictation templates.

Reprinted with permission from Allscripts Healthcare Solutions (www.allscripts.com).[9]

FIGURE   2-17

Review Dictation for Accuracy

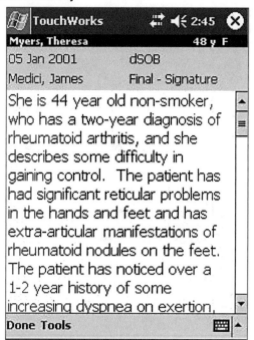

How to read this screen: Here, the transcription has been completed and the physician can access clinical documents from the PDA to provide a mobile, connected reference to the patient's chart.

Reprinted with permission from Allscripts Healthcare Solutions (www.allscripts.com).[9]

FIGURE 2-18

E/M Coder Screen From TouchWorks by Allscripts Healthcare Solutions

E/M CODER -- Web Page Dialog

E/M Coder

Setting:
- Hospital Inpatient
- Hospital Observation
- Long Term Facility
- Nursing Facility
- Outpatient

Service:
- Other Unlisted E&M
- Outpatient Consult
- Outpatient Visit
- Prev Med - Admin/Assess
- Prev Med - Group Couns
- Prev Med - Indiv Couns
- Prev Med - Other
- Prev Med Eval/Mgt
- Work/Med Disab - Dr.
- Work/Med Disab - Other

Exam Type:
- General Multi-System
- Genitourinary
- Hematologic/lymphatic/immun
- Musculoskeletal
- Neurological

Patient Status:
- NewPatient
- Established Patient

Total time spent with patient:
20 Minutes

☐ > 50% of time spent counseling / coordinating care

Documentation Levels: ▭ = Level Abstracted from Findings   ▭ = Level Set by User Override

HPI	ROS	PFSH	Overall History	EXAM	Complex of Data	Dx/Mgt	Overall Complex of MDM	Prob Risk	Tests Risk	Mgt Risk	Overall Risk
Extended (4+)	Complete (10+)	Complete (2-3 of 3)	Compreh	Compreh	Extended	Extended	High	Level 4	Level 4	Level 4	High
	Extended (2-9)		Detailed	Detailed	Moderate	Multiple	Moderate	Level 3	Level 3	Level 3	Moderate
Brief (1-3)	Pertinent (1)	Pertinent (1)	EPF	EPF	Limited	Limited	Low	Level 2	Level 2	Level 2	Low
			PF	PF	Minimal	Minimal	Minimal	Level 1	Level 1	Level 1	Minimal

E/M Code Recommendations:

Calculated from Abstracted Levels: ○ 99212 Focused H&P With Straightforward Decision Making

[Re-Calculate] **With User Override Levels:** ◉ 99213 Expanded H&P With Low Complexity Decision Making

☑ **Post Text to Current Note**   ☐ **Post Charge to Current Encounter**   [OK] [Cancel]

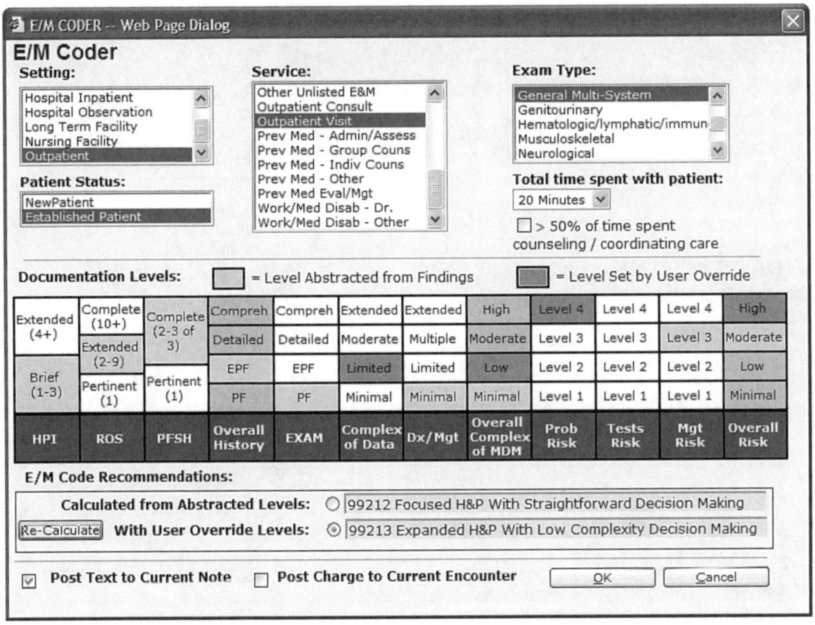

How to read this screen: Used on a desktop computer, this evaluation and management coder allows a physician to review the level of service calculated. The E/M code is automatically abstracted from the structured findings documented in the clinical note. Physicians can confirm the particular level of service abstracted or override the level selected by the system.

Reprinted with permission from Allscripts Healthcare Solutions (www.allscripts.com).[9]

FIGURE   2-19

Billing Screen From eClinicalWorks

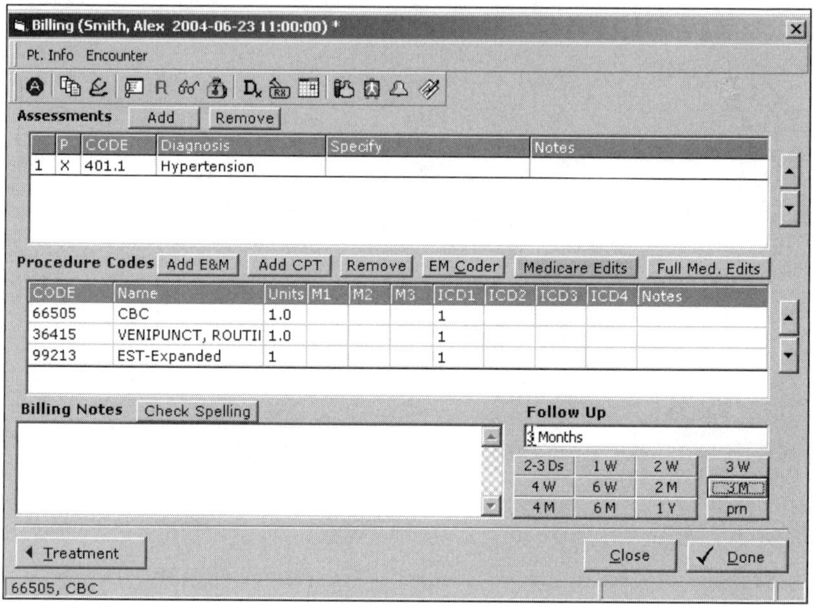

How to read this screen: The billing screen from each EMR vendor performs a specific function based on a logical sequence for capturing data. Here, the physician has entered most of the data from the patient visit, including test results and recommended follow-up exams.

Reprinted with permission from eClinicalWorks, offered online by IntegriMED (www.integrimed.com).[8]

F I G U R E 2-20

eClinicalWorks' E&M Coder. In this screen physicians can capture E&M codes.

How to read this screen: The next part of the coding process in this two-part screen set is to review the evaluation and management (E&M) coding that identifies the level of medical decision making. Ideally, the payer will reimburse the physician at the E&M coding level for this procedure.

Reprinted with permission from eClinicalWorks, offered online at IntegriMED (www.integrimed.com).[8]

Case Study: Community Care Network Nets Benefits

"One of the most common billing mistakes physicians make is that they get comfortable billing at one level for all office visits," said Kemal Erkan, Director of Blue Ox Medical Solutions, a Delaware-based business advisor for physician practices.[20] "A Level 3 claim makes them feel comfortable because they believe it will keep them out of a fraud investigation." But Erkan said that a Level 3 is not a wise billing choice when treating both the patient with cold sores and a patient recovering from double bypass surgery.

continued

"We guarantee that physicians will increase billings by at least 10% when they work with us," Erkan said. "Typical overhead for a physician practice is about 55%. When purchasing new software, our clients have to feel comfortable that their investment will help them manage or reduce that overhead."

On staff at Blue Ox are three professional financial consultants with MBAs, 10 coders working on certification, and another three certified full-time coders. Divided into departments, the Blue Ox billing and coding staff assists with data entry, charge entry, credentialing, accounts receivable, and payment posting.

The promise of enhanced billing guidance, combined with Cerner Corporation's (www.cerner.com) PowerChart Office™, seems to be the darling of Delaware and five neighboring states. Twenty-two percent of Delaware's population is serviced by the Community Care Network, a collaboration of primary care physicians, specialists, laboratories, and hospitals that share electronic patient health records on a secure Web-based format.

As a reseller for Cerner Corporation, Blue Ox formed the Community Care Network and negotiated a reduced fee for an otherwise costly EMR with EHR interoperability. Practices pay $150 per user per month. That fee includes free software upgrades every three months and a major upgrade every year.

"The real key to success is in training and implementation," Erkan said. "For a fee, we provide 12 hours of training for each user and unlimited 24-hour-a-day support for the physicians." Physician training encompasses everything from how to use a keyboard or tablet PC to how to code a specific procedure.

When implementing an EMR, sequential levels of adoption typically begin with modules that save administrative costs, such as

- Data capture and data access for electronic patient records: search, accessibility, and security
- Medical transcribing
- Electronic prescriptions
- Billing and charge capture

Once the infrastructure is in place and workforce members have moved into an electronic culture, the next module offering clinical and billing support is the Decision Support module. Decision support refers to some or all of the following:

- Most current clinical updates on new disease management techniques
- Clinical pathways and care plans
- Reminders for regulatory requirements
- Flags that duplicate documentation
- Alerts for potential medical errors

- Templates for developing evaluation and management summaries
- Billing and coding support, including dictionaries that support SNOMED-CT, ICD-9, CPT, and HCPCS codes
- Diagnostic help when patients present with yet unseen conditions
- Mobility through the practice and hospital
- Clinical consistency for new or part-time nurses
- Clinical registries
- Quality assurance, including cost and quality policies
- Cost measuring
- Capture of practice data such as patient satisfaction and clinical outcomes that demonstrate value to patients, managed care organizations, hospitals, and consumers (Some managed care plans pay bonuses to physicians who show an improvement in patient outcome with chronic conditions or deliver preventive healthcare services, such as immunizations, Pap smears, and cancer screenings.)

The following section offers guidelines on clinical decision support.

Workflow Module: Clinical Decision Support

In its book, *Crossing the Quality Chasm: A New Health System for the 21st Century*, the Institute of Medicine laid out 10 simple rules, or principles, to assist physicians in clinical decision support.[21] (These 10 principles are discussed in more detail in Chapter 1.)

Four of those 10 rules apply specifically to this module:

- Decision making should be evidence based
- Care should be customized according to patients' needs and values
- Safety should be integrated into patient care systems
- Knowledge should be shared and information should flow freely

A host of clinical decision system options are available to physicians. An EMR system that automates clinical workflow allows physicians to manage large quantities of rapidly changing health information efficiently and seamlessly.

"A clinical information system is much more a strategy than a product or an architecture," said Simon J. Samaha, MD, Vice President of Information Technology and Chief Information Officer (CIO) of the Cooper Health System in Camden, New Jersey. "I define it as a combination of clusters; one cluster will have physician order entry, result retrieval, documentation, decision support, the flowcharts, and the notes. The second is ancillary services—radiology, lab, and pharmacy; and then two new components, such as picture archiving and communications systems (PACS) and biomedical equipment."[22]

FIGURE 2-21

Clinical Decision Support in Physical Exam

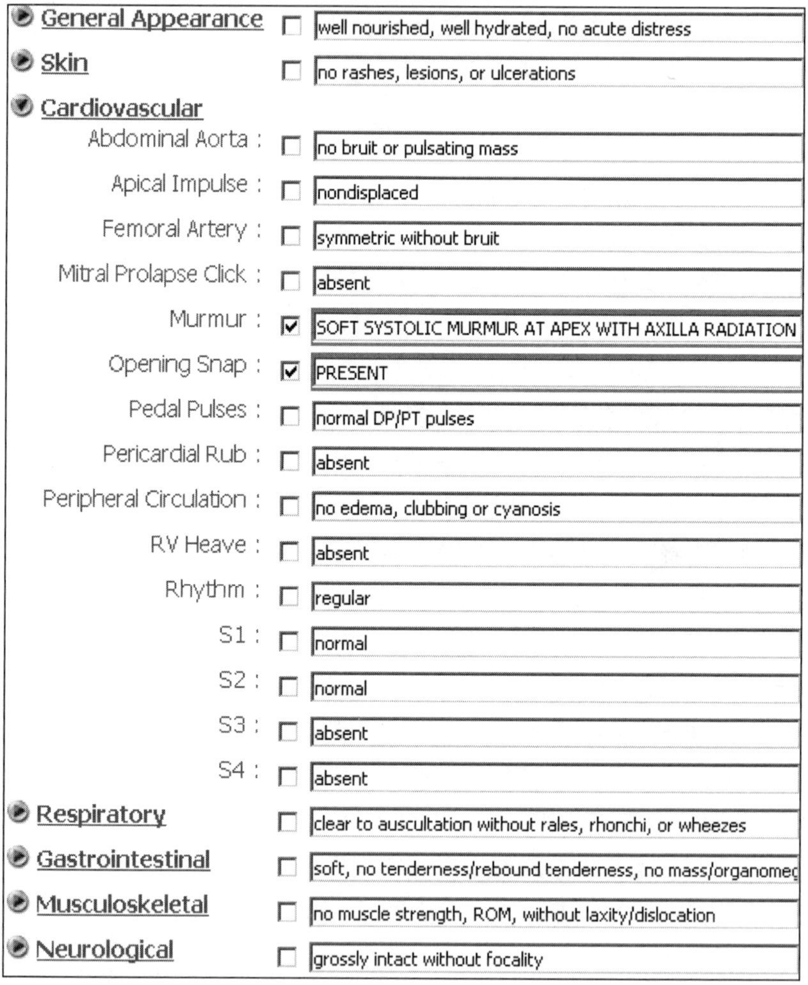

General Appearance	☐	well nourished, well hydrated, no acute distress
Skin	☐	no rashes, lesions, or ulcerations
Cardiovascular		
Abdominal Aorta :	☐	no bruit or pulsating mass
Apical Impulse :	☐	nondisplaced
Femoral Artery :	☐	symmetric without bruit
Mitral Prolapse Click :	☐	absent
Murmur :	☑	SOFT SYSTOLIC MURMUR AT APEX WITH AXILLA RADIATION
Opening Snap :	☑	PRESENT
Pedal Pulses :	☐	normal DP/PT pulses
Pericardial Rub :	☐	absent
Peripheral Circulation :	☐	no edema, clubbing or cyanosis
RV Heave :	☐	absent
Rhythm :	☐	regular
S1 :	☐	normal
S2 :	☐	normal
S3 :	☐	absent
S4 :	☐	absent
Respiratory	☐	clear to auscultation without rales, rhonchi, or wheezes
Gastrointestinal	☐	soft, no tenderness/rebound tenderness, no mass/organomeg
Musculoskeletal	☐	no muscle strength, ROM, without laxity/dislocation
Neurological	☐	grossly intact without focality

Reprinted with permission from SynaMed (www.synamed).[5]

In a physical exam, doctors evaluate symptoms and vital signs to make a diagnosis and treatment plan, based on several clinical observations. Those diagnoses can be influenced by several factors, including the patient's lifestyle, seasonal viruses, gender, and race. The software offered by SynaMed, shown in Figure 2-21, provides physicians with a framework for additional clinical inquiries based on clinical data gathered during the patient's history and physical exam. These inquiries help the physician confirm the diagnosis and treatment plan; or they may recommend additional tests if the evaluation is inconclusive.

Workflow Module: Medical Charts and Medical Transcription

Clinical workflow is anything but simple when it comes to transcription services. In the paper-based office, medical transcription usually occurs after the patient has left the office. Even when the paper process is simplified, without any regulatory privacy or security imposition, it might look like the workflow in Figure 2-22.

FIGURE 2-22

Medical Transcription Workflow in a Paper-Based Office

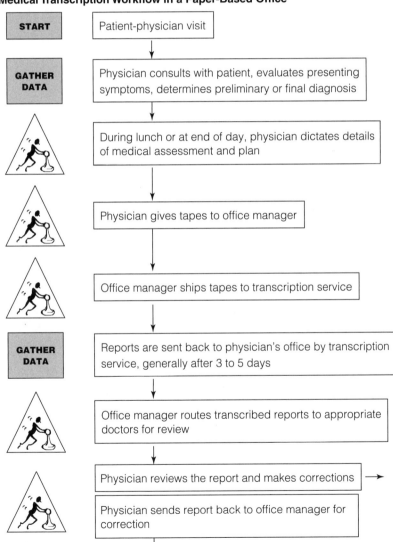

continued

FIGURE 2-22

Medical Transcription Workflow in a Paper-Based Office cont'd

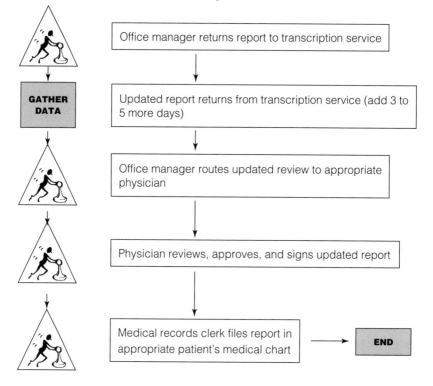

Medical transcription costs can range from $30,000 per year for a small group practice to more than $100,000 per month in a large multispecialty, multilocation practice. These are hard costs that cut into the bottom line. However, there are less obvious soft or unexpected costs as well, such as administrative staff time, shipping or delivery costs to and from the office, and time spent searching for files that may be stacked at a desk or nurse's station. When an EMR is used, medical transcription can be built from templates during the physician's physical exam and assessment, as shown in Figure 2-23. When evaluating the EMR return on investment, most vendors first point to savings received from medical transcription fees because transcription is one of the most frustrating paper shuffle exercises in the medical practice.

Prior to installing Misys Healthcare Systems in his practice, Doug Holmes, MD, an ear, nose, and throat (ENT) specialist, said he spent several years at late-night and weekend dictation, usually delivering similar information on patients with similar conditions.

FIGURE 2-23

Medical Transcription With an EMR

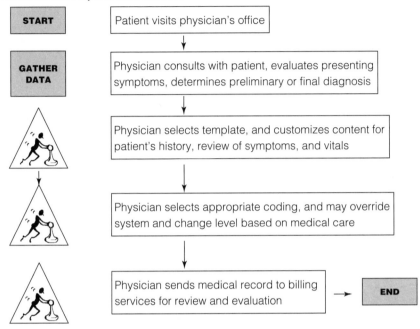

Dr Jerry Bernstein, a pediatrician in Raleigh, said parents with a sick child often return within a day or two if the child isn't showing signs of improvement. Depending on the transcription service, the patient record may or may not have been transcribed and may or may not have been returned in time for the child's repeat visit. Without the patient's history and physical exam notes, the pediatrician is dependent on the parent's accuracy when explaining the assessment and treatment plan from the previous visit.

But after switching to EMRs, both Dr Holmes and Dr Bernstein customized a short list of common diagnoses, commonly prescribed medications, and commonly used lab requests to develop a protocol, or template. With one click, the physicians can access the protocol and customize it for each patient. This information can then be used for E&M coding, eliminating the need for a transcription service. Best of all, the physicians have access to an updated medical record within 24 hours of the patient visit.

Workflow Module: Connectivity With Other Providers, Labs, and Radiology

In most practices, when a patient is referred from his or her primary care practitioner to a specialist, the message carrier is the patient. Frequently, the patient is the one who brings back results to the referring physician, if they get back to the referring physician at all. This means that the specialist is likely to obtain whatever information the patient wants to provide. Because patients tend to not want to admit they have an illness, the specialist often conducts duplicate tests or spends additional time in reevaluation. As a result, specialists often evaluate an incomplete or inaccurate medical history. The workflow in this situation consists of one set of disconnected activities after another, as shown in Figure 2-24.

Early adopters of EMRs found that data stored in one software application was often encrypted for proprietary, privacy, and security reasons. The industry-wide result could be 3,000 to 50,000 silos of patient information.[23]

It is because of these silos that Health Level Seven (HL7) has been working to adopt electronic health record standards that will enable primary care physicians, specialists, home healthcare providers, hospitals,

FIGURE   2-24

The Paper Shuffle From Provider to Referring Physician

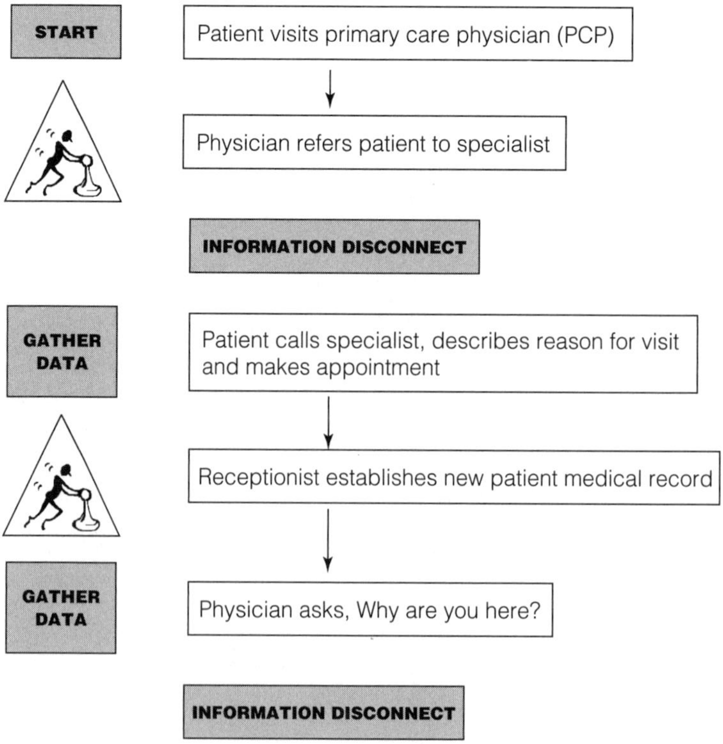

START — Patient visits primary care physician (PCP)

Physician refers patient to specialist

INFORMATION DISCONNECT

GATHER DATA — Patient calls specialist, describes reason for visit and makes appointment

Receptionist establishes new patient medical record

GATHER DATA — Physician asks, Why are you here?

INFORMATION DISCONNECT

continued

FIGURE 2-24

The Paper Shuffle From Provider to Referring Physician cont'd

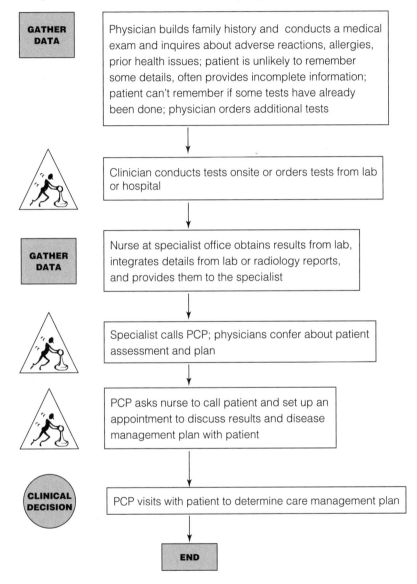

GATHER DATA — Physician builds family history and conducts a medical exam and inquires about adverse reactions, allergies, prior health issues; patient is unlikely to remember some details, often provides incomplete information; patient can't remember if some tests have already been done; physician orders additional tests

Clinician conducts tests onsite or orders tests from lab or hospital

GATHER DATA — Nurse at specialist office obtains results from lab, integrates details from lab or radiology reports, and provides them to the specialist

Specialist calls PCP; physicians confer about patient assessment and plan

PCP asks nurse to call patient and set up an appointment to discuss results and disease management plan with patient

CLINICAL DECISION — PCP visits with patient to determine care management plan

END

and ambulatory care facilities to read and react to the same patient information without the risk of exposing the patient's confidential medical files. The short- and long-term solution to interoperability is to find EMR applications that are accessible and transportable via secure Internet transactions.

STEP 4: EVALUATE THE PATIENT'S ROLE IN WORKFLOW MANAGEMENT

The one health policy issue that everyone agrees upon is that the healthcare system is badly in need of transformation. "What we have right now is the best medical talent, technology, and facilities in the world—but the system that delivers our care is badly broken," said Newt Gingrich, former Republican speaker of the House. "Democrats and Republicans should agree that moving American medicine into the twenty-first century is not only an important goal, it is also literally a matter of life and death."[24]

The transformation is in process as physicians adopt a new view toward patient involvement. Technology that works for banking, retail online sales, and manufacturing is coming to healthcare. In an era of consumer medicine and increasing safeguards on personal privacy, physicians are putting some of the responsibility for care back with the patient.

"Get the patient to do some of the administrative work for you," said Steve Malik, president and CEO of MedFusion (www.medfusion.net), a

FIGURE 2-25

Notice of Privacy Practices. Patients acknowledge receipt of Notice of Privacy Practices before submitting any confidential health information.

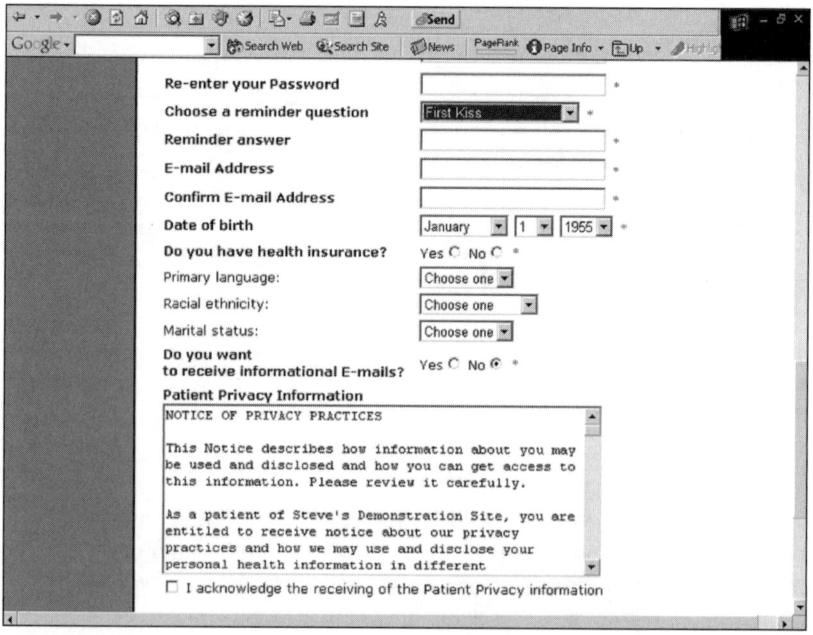

Reprinted with permission from MedFusion (www.medfusion.net).

company that builds secure Web sites for physicians who want to improve communication between their medical practices and patients.

Malik says the future of your patients' technology involvement includes some or all of the following:

■ Patient preregistration
■ Online Notice of Privacy Practices (see Figure 2-25)
■ Eligibility checks
■ Processing of bill payments (see Figure 2-26)
■ Scheduling of appointments
■ E-mail reminders to reduce no-shows
■ Prescription renewals
■ Communication of lab results (see Figure 2-27)
■ Assessment of symptoms
■ Patient education and videos
■ Virtual office visits (see Figures 2-28, 2-29, and 2-30)
■ Chronic disease management

FIGURE 2-26

Patient Online Bill Payment. Patients can review and pay their balances online through your merchant account.

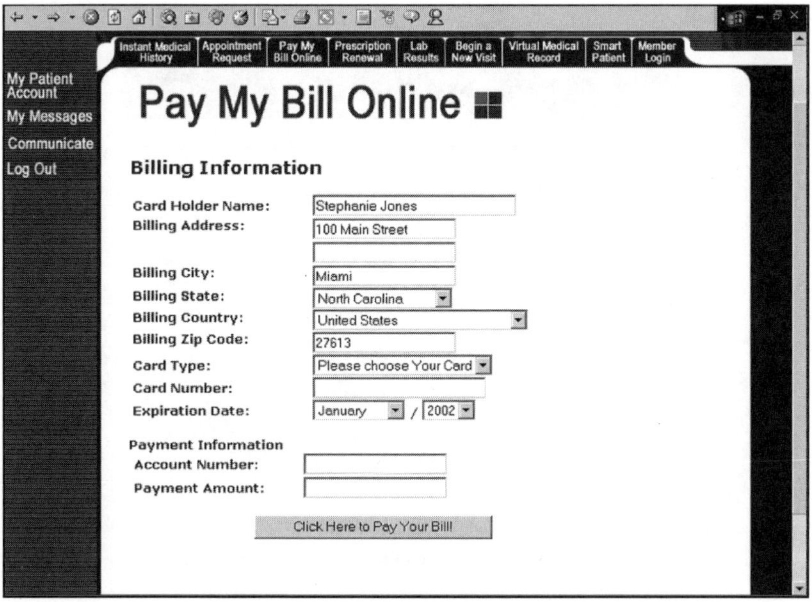

Reprinted with permission from MedFusion (www.medfusion.net).

FIGURE 2-27

Lab Results. You determine whether to provide lab results online or call the patient directly through this lab reporting process.

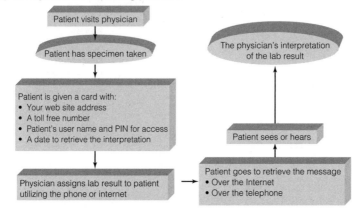

Reprinted with permission from MedFusion (www.medfusion.net).

FIGURE 2-28

Virtual Office Visit, Part 1: Physician's View. All communication must be encrypted and secure. Physician logs into secure area to begin the process.

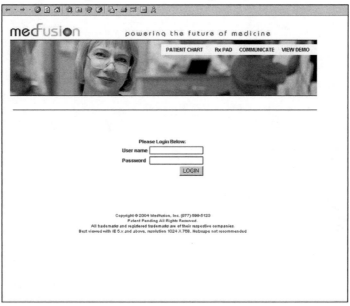

Reprinted with permission from MedFusion (www.medfusion.net).

FIGURE 2-29

Virtual Office Visit, Part 2: Physician's View. The Communication Center tells the physician how many patients are waiting in the "New patient(s)" section.

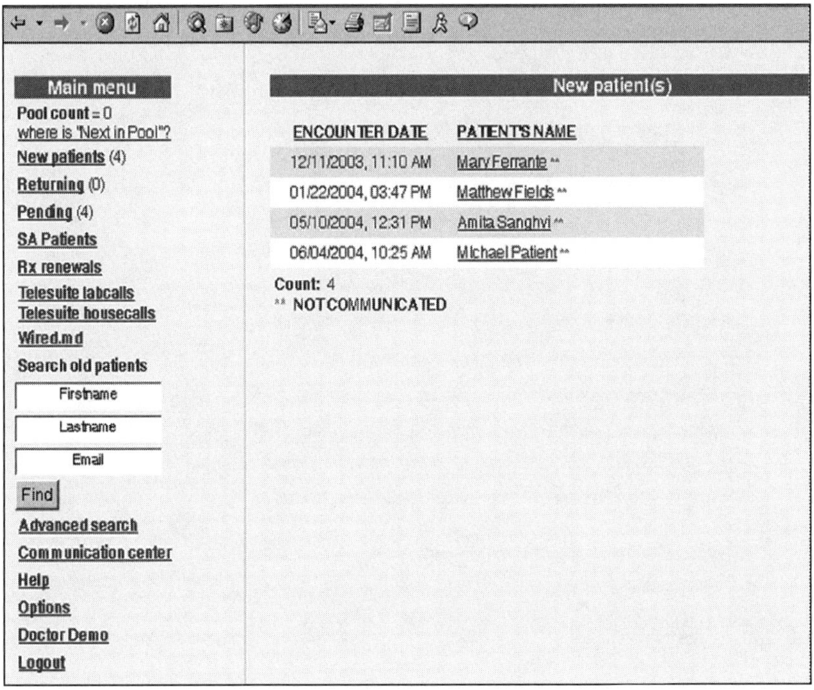

Reprinted with permission from MedFusion (www.medfusion.net).

FIGURE 2-30

Virtual Office Visit, Part 3: Physician's View. The physician selects patient and views patient's request.

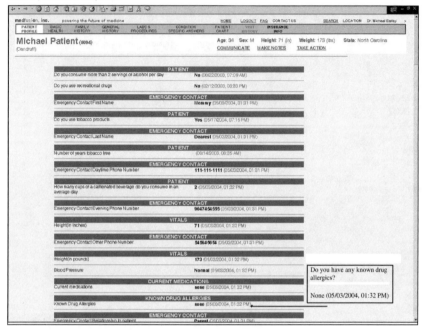

STEP 5: BRIDGE THE WORKFLOW GAP FROM PAPER TO ELECTRONIC MEDICAL RECORD

From the flowcharts presented in this chapter, you can see that the move to an EMR with EHR interoperability is a significant cultural and workflow change for the medical staff. Without planning, analyzing, and communicating details about the work process, your current EMR components may not be understood and will fail, an unpleasant end to a significant investment.

You won't be able to go totally paperless until labs, hospitals, and other clinicians go paperless—an ambitious goal that all branches of the federal government hope to achieve by 2014.[25] In Chapter 4, we show you how to implement a hybrid EHR, one that blends paper-based functions with electronic functions.

SUMMARY

In the first two chapters, we provided you with an overview of EMRs and we examined workflow in a paper-based office and what it will look like in an electronic environment. In both chapters, we referenced EHR standards that are in various stages of testing and evaluation. In Chapter 3, we provide you with an in-depth analysis of LOINC, SNOMED-CT, and CHI, clinical data sets that support the components of the EHR. In Chapter 4, we describe the functional descriptors of the Draft Standard for Trial Use (DTSU) electronic health record (EHR) that HL7 began piloting for 2 years, starting in July 2004.

ENDNOTES

1. Medical Records Institute Fifth Annual Survey of EHR Trends and Usage. Available at: www.medrecinst.org.

2. Definitions provided by *HL7 Glossary of Terms.* (Health Level Seven, Inc; 2002.)

3. In this and other examples in this chapter, we use the terms *workforce* and *staff* interchangeably. Workforce has a certain connotation with respect to protected health information (PHI) under the Privacy and Security Rule provisions of HIPAA. By using the shorter word, *staff,* in the examples for economy of space, we in no way lessen workforce responsibilities and accountabilities for safeguarding PHI.

4. Sample screen provided by A4 Health Systems. A4 Health Systems ensures that any names used in its screens are fictitious and used for demonstration purposes only. For an online demonstration, go to www.a4healthsystems. com/contact.asp.

5. Any reference to physician or patient is strictly fictional and for demonstration purposes only. They are not intended to bear any resemblance to any person, living or deceased.

6. Sample screen provided by SynaMed. SynaMed ensures that any names used in its screens are fictitious and used for demonstration purposes only. For an online demonstration, go to www.synamed.com.

7. To learn more about IntegriMED or for a demonstration of eClinicalWorks online, go to www.integrimed.com.

8. Sample screen provided by eClinicalWorks, which is available online by IntegriMED at www.integrimed.com. eClinicalWorks and IntegriMED ensure that any names used in its screens are fictitious and used for demonstration purposes only. For an online demonstration, go to www.integrimed.com.

9. Sample screen provided by Allscripts Healthcare Solutions. Allscripts ensures that any names used in its screens are fictitious and used for demonstration purposes only. For an online demonstration, go to: www.allscripts.com

10. To download a free copy of Adobe® Reader®, software for viewing and print-ing portable document format (PDF) documents, go to www.adobe.com/ products/acrobat/readstep2.html.

11. Centers for Medicare and Medicaid Services, 42 CFR Parts 405 and 414, Medicare program: changes to Medicare payment for drugs and physician fee schedule payments for calendar year 2004, Interim Final Rule. *Federal Register.* 2004;69:1083–1267. (A PDF version of the regulation is available on the CMS Web site at www.cms.hhs.gov/mmu.)

12. Hensley S. Medicare move likely to benefit costliest drugs. *Wall Street Journal.* February 24, 2004:B1.

13. Twight C. Medicare's origin: the economics and politics of dependency. *Cato J.* 1997;16(3). Available at: www.cato.org/pubs/journal/cj16n3-3.html.

14. Section 108: Grants to Physicians to Implement Electronic Prescription Drug Programs. Medicare Prescription Drug Improvement and Modernization Act of 2003:107-108.

15. HHS launches new efforts to promote paperless health care system [news release]. Washington, DC: US Department of Health and Human Resources; July 1, 2003. Available at: www.hhs.gov/news/press/2003press/20030701. html. (For a discussion of the electronic prescription as a component of the electronic health record, see *HIPAA Transactions: A Nontechnical Guide for Health Care* by Edward D. Jones III and Carolyn P. Hartley. [AMA Press; 2004].)

16. Subsections (3)(A) and (3)(B). Medicare Prescription Drug Improvement and Modernization Act of 2003:23.

17. Subsection (5)(A). Medicare Prescription Drug Improvement and Modernization Act of 2003:25.

18. Jones E. Medicare comes of age. *Physician's e-Health Report.* March/April 2004.

19. American Academy of Family Physicians. Take the EHR readiness assessment. Leawood, Kan: AAFP; Sept., 2004. In the initial survey, 877 respondents in 21 chapters responded to the survey.

20. E&M billing levels from 1 to 5 are used to describe the complexity of the physician's or nurse's involvement in patient evaluation and care management. The level results in the corresponding amount reimbursed by the payer to the physician. A level 3 is midrange, with 1 being the lowest and 5 the most complex. A practice management consultant should call into question one physician's consistent use of level 3.

21. Committee on Quality of Health Care in America. *Crossing the Quality Chasm: A New Health System for the 21st Century.* Washington, DC: National Academy Press; 2001.

22. *Straight Talk,* presented by *Modern Healthcare* and PricewaterhouseCoopers; discussion held on January 9, 2003 at *Modern Healthcare's* Chicago headquarters, moderated by Charles S. Lauer. A transcript of that discussion is available at: http://healthcare.pwc.com/st200201.html.

23. "When Buying an EMR, Avoid Getting Bruised by Technology," quoting John Quinn, principal, Capgemini, in *Physician's e-Health Report,* April/May 2004. Available online at: www.physiciansehr.com.

24. Gingrich G, Kennedy P. Operating in a vacuum. *New York Times.* May 3, 2004.

25. Footnote from a speech by David Brailer, MD, PhD, national coordinator for health information technology, July 21, 2004.

Making the Purchase

Forrester Research analysts indicate that beginning in 2005, sales of electronic medical records (EMRs) to small practices will surpass those to larger practices.[1] The explanation offered by the report's authors is that EMRs have become more stable; they've been accepted by early adopters; and more EMR companies are reaching out to small and midsize physician practices. This amounts to too many sellers chasing a set number of practices.[2]

What should you expect to pay for an EMR, and how soon will you experience a return on investment? Who should be involved in the buying decision and how will you know if you're buying something that actually works?

Buying an EMR system has been compared to purchasing a car. However, in researching and writing this book, we've learned the purchase of an EMR is much more complex. A car will get you where you want to be with some degree of style. An EMR, however, affects everyone in your practice as well as your billing and payments, your scheduling, your clinical decision making, and your communication strategies with your patients. And most important, it influences your office culture.

For these reasons, we have identified 12 steps that will keep everyone in the workforce involved in the EMR decision—from the president of the practice to the front line. This chapter guides you through this 12-step process and helps you make a decision that's right for your budget, your workflow, and the people in your practice.

WHAT YOU WILL LEARN IN THIS CHAPTER

- How to budget for an EMR/EHR system that is interoperable with providers, payers, and patients
- The look of your implementation dream team
- The 12-step process to select the right system for your organization
- What to include in your request for proposal
- How to score vendors by function and usability

- The patient's role in your EHR/EMR decision
- How to negotiate the deal
- Why commitment is necessary for success

Key Terms

Application Service Provider (ASP): A third-party entity that distributes software and software-based services and solutions to a large geographical area over the Internet from a central data center.

Certification Commission for Healthcare Information Technology (CCHIT): A certification authority formed by three healthcare organizations (American Health Information Management Association [AHIMA], Healthcare Information and Management Systems Society [HIMSS], and National Alliance for Health Information Technology) that works to create an efficient, impartial, and trusted mechanism to certify ambulatory electronic health records and other healthcare information technology (IT) products.[3]

Request for Proposal (RFP): The beginning of the software selection process by which a prospective software purchaser specifics details of the system required.

Before making an EMR or electronic health record (EHR) system purchase, first evaluate what is already in place. Most physician practices use practice management (PM) software that organizes the practice's administrative activities. You probably use the PM software to schedule patients, track billing and payments, and store patient contact and insurance information. But, as discussed in Chapters 1 and 2, it was rare that PM software from one vendor was interoperable with another vendor's software, resulting in significant communication delays, poor integration of clinical data, and increased administrative costs.

Electronic medical record vendors have known for years about the move to interoperability, and have been working with committees such as Health Level Seven (HL7) to upgrade their PM software for interoperability. Unless your current vendor's PM software does not meet your needs, we recommend that you include and compare your current vendor in your step-by-step search for a new EHR system.

In the following discussion of steps a practice should undertake in evaluating electronic record systems, we focus on decisions relating to EMR decision-making, many of which apply to EHR system decision-making as well. In Chapter 6, we describe EHR systems in detail, focusing on functional descriptors of HL7's EHR Draft Standard for Trial Use (DSTU).

STEP 1: ESTABLISH YOUR BUDGET FOR AN ELECTRONIC HEALTH RECORD SYSTEM

We've moved the bottom line to the top of this chapter because we know the structure and cost of an EHR system will influence your buying decision.

There are two technology approaches when considering an EHR:

- A software licensing fee per user or per physician
  — Prices range from $15,000 to $50,000 per physician, although we've seen them as high as $75,000 to $100,000 for a solo specialty practice.
- An application service provider (ASP) plan
  — Prices range from $99/month to $700/month per user or per physician.
  — Many ASP vendors also impose monthly fees for specific transactions. Some ASP-based vendors take a percentage of any fees collected from an online virtual medical office visit. Others may collect a fee each time you file a claim for reimbursement.

Regarding this wide range in software costs, Mark Anderson writes in *Information Technology Trends and Solutions 2004 EMR Survey*, "Software costs alone per physician vary by company and are not necessarily related to top functionality."[4] In other words, the costliest EMRs might not necessarily offer the best solution for a physician practice. To make a purchasing decision that you can live with, we recommend the following:

- Identify the functions, training, and implementation options that are most important to you and your workforce.
- Follow the selection and purchasing steps in this chapter so that you don't spend $75,000 when $5,000 to $10,000 a year would fit into your budget.
- Use the information you've gathered to select three or four top vendors. Through several processes of elimination, you'll likely end up with a choice of one or two vendors that complement your workload, your budget, and implementation expectations.

STEP 2: ESTABLISH YOUR IMPLEMENTATION DREAM TEAM

In large physician practices and hospital networks, 39% of respondents in the 2004 Healthcare Information and Management Systems Society (HIMSS) annual survey said that it was the chief information officer (CIO) who made the decision on which EHR system to purchase.[5] However, as illustrated in Figure 3-1, 24% indicated the chief executive officer (CEO) made the final decision, 17% said it was the chief financial officer (CFO), and 5% indicated the chief medical officer (CMO) got the honors.

Parlay those statistics into the physician's practice and the dream team translates into the following participants:

- Physician managing partner or practice owner (CEO)
- Financial advisor/practice management consultant (CFO)

FIGURE 3-1

Who Is the EHR Decision Maker?

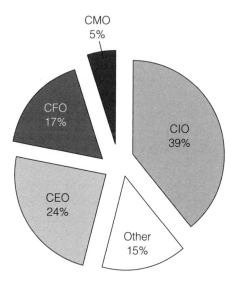

Source: 15th Annual HIMSS Leadership Survey sponsored by Superior Consultant Company.

- Billing and coding workforce member (CFO)
- Office manager (CIO)
- Scheduler (CIO)
- Medical records workforce member (CIO)
- Physician partner (CMO)
- Nurse practitioner (While none of the hospitals indicated a chief nursing officer [CNO] made the buying decision, we strongly advise that a member of the nursing staff be part of your implementation team.)

STEP 3: ENGAGE THE TEAM BUT BE CLEAR ABOUT WHO WILL MAKE THE FINAL DECISION

As with most management actions, you must control the decision process so that it doesn't get out of hand. You can preview many appealing systems with available options that appear to be what you need, but they are of no value if they're not right for your practice.

For example, you may find tablet PCs or handheld prescribing to be time-savers, while another physician practice may consider them to be gimmicky.

Appoint one person to be the "EHR champion," or someone who will lead the effort and inspire the practice to keep moving through EHR implementation. Each vendor we interviewed told us a successful EHR implementation contained three common elements:

- At least one physician champion
- Role-based training customized for physicians and workforce members
- Vendor-integrated information technology (IT) implementation with an outside consultant implementing the EHR

As you enter the EHR adoption process, watch for anxiety among workforce members. Some people are hesitant to get excited about EHRs or may even offer negative input because they fear their jobs will be eliminated.

There's no doubt about it, the decision to move into an electronic environment will definitely change the paper-based work environment. Most physician practices choose to retrain employees, but it is up to practice leadership on how to proceed with reassigning and retraining workforce members.

Early EHR adopters tell us that it's rare that a medical office reduces its staff. Instead, workforce members assume new job responsibilities because electronic workflow processes may allow your practice to see additional patients. You may decide to maintain the same patient census, in which case, through attrition, vacated positions may not need to be refilled.

STEP 4: PRIORITIZE WHAT YOU WANT

You probably want an EHR system that saves time, improves patient safety, improves cash flow, assists in clinical decision support, reduces rejected claims, and gets you home early to your family. These are results of an efficient EHR system. To obtain these results, identify functions that help you achieve your outcomes. Table 3-1 presents a checklist of priorities.

T A B L E 3-1

Checklist for Prioritizing EHR System Functions

Place a check mark in areas that are top, middle, or low priority for you.

Function	How It Is Used in the Practice	Top	Middle	Low
Views patient information	Review patient's symptoms or chief complaints, medication list, test results, other clinical documentation			
Gathers data	Build electronic patient charts that are searchable and downloadable. Build a patient's chart from customizable templates			

continued

TABLE 3-1

Checklist for Prioritizing EHR System Functions cont'd

Function	How It Is Used in the Practice	Priority		
		Top	Middle	Low
Compile data	Pull together patient or practice census and histories and graph or map this information for analysis			
Clinical decision support	Assist in evaluating, diagnosing, and reviewing acute or chronic diseases			
Interoperability with other systems	Interact with internal practice management software, billing, and coding. Provide your practice with information on most profitable payers			
Search capabilities	Query your database for reports on clinical issues and costs			
Patient management	Manage an individual patient's acute and chronic diseases and conditions			
Practice marketing	Inform your practice of types of services you perform most often. Provide analyses on your patients' clinical commonalities, referral base, patient census			
Standardization	Standardize disease management goals for patient groups within your practice			
Billing and coding	Establish internal checks and balances and tie International Classification of Diseases (ICD) and Current Procedural Terminology (CPT®) codes to details of the patient encounter; integrate evaluation and management (E&M) coding; and maintain databases of Systematized Nomenclature of Medicine-Clinical Terms (SNOMED-CT), Logical Observation Identifiers Names and Codes (LOINC), and Healthcare Common Procedure Coding System (HCPCS) codes			
Order entry	Order labs, images, other nonmedications			
e-Prescribing	Authorize and manage prescription refills. Access formulary information. Route new prescriptions online to pharmacy			

continued

TABLE 3-1

Checklist for Prioritizing EHR System Functions cont'd

Function	How It Is Used in the Practice	Priority		
		Top	**Middle**	**Low**
Communication	Communicate online with patients and colleagues			
Compliance	Provide built-in compliance and regulatory guidance			
Clinical trials	Conduct research, registry, and clinical trial activities			
Patient interaction	Incorporate information originating from the patient and from medical and patient devices			

This checklist is an important document to reference when selecting an EMR vendor. It also can be used to help you plan your implementation strategy discussed in Chapter 4.

STEP 5: ASSIGN FACT-FINDING DUTIES AND RESPONSIBILITIES TO EACH MEMBER OF THE IMPLEMENTATION TEAM

Now that you have an idea of what's important to your practice, use the top- and middle-priority lists generated from Table 3-1 to identify which vendors provide the functions you want in an EHR.

■ **Talk to your colleagues.** Ask fellow physicians about which EHR systems are used in their practices and what they like/dislike about their systems. Ask each practice how much training is available to the physician and staff, and who performed the training. Ask how long it took your colleague's office to implement the EHR system. Ask if they adopted the entire EHR system at once or if they implemented it in modules. Ask what they would do differently.

EHR Tip: Guard against making a decision because another physician likes a particular EHR system. Often, EHR systems are customized for practice, specialty, and size.

■ **Hold off on purchasing new hardware until you've selected your EHR system.** In the early adoption stages, physician groups purchased and implemented hardware, software, and consulting services, but several vendors reported that the return rate on the software was substantial. Inadequate knowledge of the practice, poor or incomplete implementation, and irregular training were often cited as reasons for the EMR returns. Today, most physicians are remaining with the EHR vendor for a long time, so hold off on purchasing any new computers, printers, data storage units, handheld devices, and so forth until you find out what is required from the EHR vendor your select.

■ **Evaluate EHR systems that are compatible with your specialty and practice size.** In its *Information Technology Trends and Solutions: 2004 Summary Report,* the AC Group ranked the top EMR applications by asking 5,155 functional questions in 27 categories and four methods of operations.[4] (The summary of that report is available in Appendix C of this book and online at www.acgroup.org.) Four charts from that report are recreated here in Tables 3-2, 3-3, 3-4, and 3-5. These tables identify the overall score and ranking of EHRs for physician practices in four categories:

— 100+ physicians

— 15 to 99 physicians

— five to 15 physicians

— one to four physicians

TABLE 3-2

Large Practices: Greater Than 100 Physicians*

Overall Ranking	Vendor	Desktop	EMR Ranking	EHR Ranking	Overall Score
1	NextGen Healthcare Systems	95.0%	5	5	37
2	Allscripts Healthcare Solutions	92.9%	5	4	37
3	SynaMed	89.7%	4	5	24
4	iMedica Corporation	89.2%	4	4	26
5	Physician Micro Systems, Inc	83.9%	4	3	30
6	Epic Systems	81.0%	4	4	30
7	Medical Communication Systems	80.8%	4	4	23
8	GE Medical	74.1%	3	1	29
9	A4 Health Systems	73.9%	3	1	28

* For larger practices with over 150 physicians, the top applications are from NextGen Healthcare Systems (95%) and Allscripts Healthcare Solutions (92.9%). Five additional vendors, SynaMed (89.7%), iMedica Corporation (89.2%), Physician Micro Systems (83.9%), Epic Systems (81.0%), and Medical Communication Systems (80.8%), scored four stars in the EMR functionality rating. NextGen and Allscripts received the highest overall point ranking once you consider company size, client base, end-user satisfaction, and price.

Reprinted with permission from AC Group, Inc.

T A B L E 3-3

Midsize Practices: 15 to 99 Physicians*

Overall Ranking	Vendor	Desktop	EMR Ranking	EHR Ranking	Overall Score
1	NextGen Healthcare Systems	95.0%	5	5	37
2	Allscripts Healthcare Solutions	92.9%	5	4	37
3	SynaMed	89.7%	4	5	24
4	iMedica Corporation	89.2%	4	4	26
5	Physician Micro Systems, Inc	83.9%	4	3	30
6	eClinicalworks	81.9%	4	4	29
7	MedInformatics	80.9%	4	1	25
8	Medical Communication Systems	80.8%	4	4	23

* For larger practices between 15 and 99 physicians, the top applications are from NextGen Healthcare Systems (95%) and Allscripts Healthcare Solutions (92.9%). Six additional vendors, SynaMed (89.7%), iMedica Corporation (89.2%), Physician Micro Systems (83.9%), eClinical- works (81.3%), MedInformatics (80.9%), and Medical Communication Systems (80.8%) scored four stars in the EMR functionality rating. Meridian EMR, MedInformatics, A4 Health Systems, and GE Medical received three stars. NextGen and Allscripts received the highest overall point ranking once you consider company size, client base, end-user satisfaction, and price.

Reprinted with permission from AC Group, Inc.

T A B L E 3-4

Small Practices: Five to 15 Physicians*

Overall Ranking	Vendor	Desktop	Rating	EHR	Overall Score
1	NextGen Healthcare Systems	95.0%	5	5	37
2	Allscripts Healthcare Solutions	92.9%	5	4	37
3	SynaMed	89.7%	4	5	24
4	iMedica Corporation	89.2%	4	4	26
5	Bond Technologies	88.1%	4	5	24
6	Physician Micro Systems, Inc	83.9%	4	3	30
7	eClinicalworks	81.9%	4	4	29
8	MedInformatics	80.9%	4	1	25

continued

TABLE 3-4

Small Practices: Five to 15 Physicians* cont'd

Overall Ranking	Vendor	Desktop	Rating	EHR	Overall Score
9	Medical Communication Systems	80.8%	4	4	23
10	JMJ Technologies	78.9%	3	1	22
11	Praxis EMR	77.2%	3	1	25
12	Meridian EMR	76.8%	3	1	15
13	GE Medical	74.1%	3	1	29
14	A4 Health Systems	73.9%	3	1	28

* For smaller vendors with five to 15 physicians the top applications remain the same as the midsized practices. Two new vendors entered this category: Bond Technologies (88.1%) and JMJ Technologies (78.9%). Many of these vendors do not actively market to this size of practice; however, all will provide a bid if requested.

Reprinted with permission from AC Group, Inc.

TABLE 3-5

Small Practices: One to four Physicians*

Overall Ranking	Vendor	Desktop	Rating	EHR	Overall Score
1	SynaMed	89.7%	4	5	24
2	Bond Technologies	88.1%	4	5	24
3	Physician Micro Systems, Inc	83.9%	4	3	30
4	eClinicalworks	81.9%	4	4	29
5	Medinformatics	80.9%	4	1	25
6	Medical Communication Systems	80.8%	4	4	23
7	JMJ Technologies	78.9%	3	1	22
8	Praxis EMR	77.2%	3	1	25
9	Meridian EMR	76.8%	3	1	15
10	A4 Health Systems	73.9%	3	1	28
11	Greenway Medical	73.7%	3	NA	18

* For smaller practices with less than five physicians, SynaMed (89.7%), Bond Technologies (88.1%), Physician Micro Systems (83.9%), and eClinicalworks (81.9%) received four stars with more than 80% of the current requirements. Physician Micro Systems and eClinicalworks received the highest overall point ranking once you consider company size, client base, end-user satisfaction, and price. Medinformatics (80.9%), JMJ Technologies (78.9%), Praxis EMR (77.2%), Meridian EMR (76.8%), A4 Health Systems (73.9%), and Greenway Medical (73.7%) rounded the top 10 EMR vendor applications for the small physician office.

Reprinted with permission from AC Group, Inc.

This ranking is important because it coincides with the customer profile most likely to correspond with the complexity of the software. Vendors that sell software to practices with more than 100 physicians may have a scaled-down version of the software for practices with fewer than five physicians per practice. (Vendors listed in Tables 3-2, 3-3, 3-4, and 3-5 are not endorsed by either the authors or the publisher, but are provided for you as a resource.)

- **Attend a trade show**. A state medical association conference is a good place to invite EMR vendors to display their software. Tell them you are in the inquiry stage and ask if they will be at a trade show near you.

- **Request an online demonstration**. Most vendors have developed fairly sophisticated online EMR demonstrations. In most cases, you'll have to register to see the demonstration, which means you're likely to get a follow-up phone call. But when it comes to EMRs, you'll want to talk to several companies. To view several free demonstrations from one location, consult www.physiciansehr.com, and select "Demo Depot" from the left-hand menu.

- **Develop a short list and a long list**. As with any selection process, decision makers develop a short list of the most likely candidates and a longer list of potential candidates (examples are provided in Tables 3-6 and 3-7). Limit the short list to two or three vendors, but keep in mind that as the demand for EHR systems increases, it may take a long time before a vendor comes to your practice, unless you are geographically close to a sales office.

STEP 6: DEVELOP A REQUEST FOR PROPOSAL AND SUBMIT IT TO THREE OR FOUR VENDORS

Call the vendors on your short list. Tell them you'd like to send them a request for proposal (RFP) and to whom it should be addressed.

TABLE 3-6

Short List of Most Likely Candidates

Name of Vendor and Contact Info	Online Demonstration Web Site Address	What You Like About This EHR System

TABLE 3-7

Long List of Potential Candidates

Name of Vendor and Contact Info	Reason for Not Making the Short List	What You Like About This EHR System

Provide a 30-day deadline for responses and stick to that deadline. At the end of 30 days, you'll know what companies can deliver on time and what companies are interested in working with you, and you'll have an approximate budget for the services you require. An RFP might look something like Figure 3-2.

FIGURE 3-2

Sample Request for Proposal for a Small to Midsize Physician Practice*

SAMPLE REQUEST FOR PROPOSAL

FOR EMR/EHR System

(Date of Proposal)

REQUESTED BY:

Name of Practice

Contact Person

Address, City, State, Zip

Phone/Fax

E-mail, if appropriate

---

1. General information

All proposals to be considered must be submitted on or before (*time, time zone*) on (*day, month, date, year*) to (*name of person, address, city, state, zip*). Any questions about the proposal may be directed to the attention of (*name, title, telephone number*).

Proposals may be submitted electronically on or before designated time at (*e-mail address*). If you are submitting electronically and by mail, please indicate this in your proposal: "Via e-mail and USPS."

The practice reserves the right to contact any Proposer if the practice needs information clarified. The practice also reserves the right to conduct due diligence research by contacting current and past customers of the Proposer, and to use other sources to obtain information about the Proposer.

Proposers are encouraged to present additional information not requested in this RFP if you believe it will make your EMR the best choice for our practice.

After reading the proposals, three EMR vendors will be selected to make a presentation to the review committee during the afternoon of (*day, month, date, year*).

2. Background information about the practice

(*Briefly describe your practice: your specialty, geographic area served, total staff, approximate patient load*)

Anticipated users

Number of physicians   _____

Number of nurses   _____

Number of workforce support   _____

Total number of anticipated users   _____

To view several free demonstrations from one location, consult www.physiciansehr.com, and select "Demo Depot" from the left-hand menu.

Existing hardware configuration list

(*List, by make, model, and year purchased, servers, printers, workstations, etc, that the practice uses to support its software programs*)

Existing software capabilities

(*List Practice Management and/or Billing software you are currently using and [a] want to continue to use or [b] would change if an alternative proved better, faster, less expensive.*)

continued

Web access *(indicate by checking what you use in the office)*

Broadband   ____

DSL   ____

Dial-up   ____

Secure Network   ____

3. Confidentiality

Information provided by the EMR vendor to the practice will be kept confidential and will not be shared with competing vendors.

4. The proposal

The purpose of this solicitation is to seek a commercial electronic health record management system that will replace or enhance the current clinical and practice information management systems used by this practice. (*Name of Practice*) believes a robust information system is essential for it to successfully compete in the practice of (*specialty*).

This solicitation contains eight response areas:

- Functional requirements

- Training and implementation requirements

- Technical requirements

- Technical support

- Strategic partners

- Market presence

- Privacy and security safeguards

- Interoperability

A. Functional requirements

How does your EMR meet our prioritized list of functional requirements? (*Adjust according to your list of priorities.*)

Patient scheduling

Patient registration

Patient interoperability

System-wide integration

Medical records

Patient case management

Patient billing

Billing forms and reports

Third-party billing

Managed care

Laboratory interface

Pharmacy management

Data inquiry and report generation[†]

B. Training and implementation requirements

Describe your implementation and training services.
What is the length of implementation from acceptance to "go-live?"

C. Technical requirements

Based on the background information described in section 2 above, will your software meet or exceed our existing technology?

D. Technical support and maintenance

Describe the technical support we should expect from your company.

Provide sample content from your user's manual.

Do you have user groups or forums?

How often do you upgrade the system?

Who decides when I need system enhancements?

How often do you schedule normal system upgrades?

Are upgrades free or for a fee?

E. Describe your relationships with strategic partners

What portion of the EMR you would provide for us is dependent upon the success of a strategic partner? Describe any relationships with strategic partners that may provide software as part of your EMR or EHR system software; so-called middle-ware.

continued

F. Presence in the marketplace

How many concurrent user licenses have you sold?

How many of your staff are involved in product development and training?

What percentage of your revenues do you devote to research and development?

What's the average size of practice that purchases your EMR?

What are your revenue projections for this year?

G. Privacy and security

Describe your privacy and security safeguards.

What is your company's approach to HIPAA compliance?

H. Interoperability

How many sites have you interfaced to the client's practice management system?

How does your system connect to labs, hospitals, home health agencies, etc, locally and in other areas?

5. Biographic details

Please provide biographic details about your company executives, including how long they have been in the field of health information technology.

6. Budget

Please provide a budget for your EMR system, including user's fees, implementation, technical support and training fees, upgrade fees, and any incidental charges that are routinely requested by physician offices of our size and specialty.

7. Right to accept or reject

Our practice reserves the right to select one or more, or none of the proposals submitted. We also reserve the right to accept or reject all or parts of proposals received.

8. Selection criteria

Our decision will be based on:

- Relevance to our practice size, specialty, and function
- Implementation plan, technical support, training, and customer service
- Cost

---

9. References

Please provide name, telephone number, and e-mail address of three references of practices similar in size and specialty mix to ours that our practice may contact.

10. Thank you

We realize this is a busy time for EMR companies and wish to thank you in advance for the effort you'll put into responding to our request. We regret that we are unable to accept any responses by phone. But please call us at (*telephone number*) if you have any questions.

---

* This RFP is for demonstration purposes and is not meant to be used or relied upon as legal advice. Please contact the attorney for your practice for such legal advice. Items in italics are for you to customize.

† This functional list was adapted from the sample RFP for an EMR, developed by the Bureau of Primary Health Care, April 7, 2004, as part of the eHealth Initiative. The full RFP is available online at: http://ccbh.ehealthinitiative.org/communities/community.aspx?Section=108&Category=164&Document=216.

Reprinted with permission from Physicians EHR, LLC (www.physiciansehr.com).

STEP 7: DEVELOP A SCORECARD AND RATE THE VENDORS ON YOUR SHORT LIST

Once you've received responses from your RFPs, you'll want to evaluate the content. All EMRs are not created equal, but try to be as fair as possible in this evaluation. Table 3-8 offers a scorecard to help you in the evaluation process.

T A B L E 3-8

Scorecard for Vendor Selection

Area of Interest	Vendor 1	Vendor 2	Vendor 3	Comments
	Scoring: 1 = low; 5 = high			
	Functionality			
View and edit daily schedule				
Patient registration Interoperable with other providers and patients				

continued

TABLE 3-8

Scorecard for Vendor Selection cont'd

Area of Interest	Vendor 1	Vendor 2	Vendor 3	Comments
	Scoring: 1 = low; 5 = high			
System-wide integration of administrative and clinical functionality				
Medical records and charting				
Patient case management				
Clinical decisions support				
Usability				
Patient billing				
Billing forms and reports				
Third-party billing				
Laboratory interface				
Pharmacy management				
Data entry and reports				
Marketing reports				
Total				
Average (divide by 15)				
User Friendly				
Input information in variety of methods (personal data assistants [PDAs], wireless, tablet PCs, mouse, stylus, touch screen)				
EMR customized for our practice				
Nontechnical (screens are understandable, and reflect our practice's workflow)				
EHR can be successfully integrated with other systems				
Remote accessibility to practice's database of medical records				

continued

TABLE 3-8

Scorecard for Vendor Selection cont'd

Area of Interest	Vendor 1	Vendor 2	Vendor 3	Comments
	Scoring: 1 = low; 5 = high			
Graphics and images (stores, exchanges, and transmits images, graphics capabilities)				
Screen appearance (you could look at and work with this screen repeatedly during the workday)				
Compatibility (used by clinical and administrative workforce members)				
Data are retrievable and readable if we change EHR vendors (Note: this can be a deal-breaker for a practice if not guaranteed in writing!)				
Doctors will use chosen EMR (Note: investment in EMR will not provide ROI if it does not reflect workflow of physicians in practice)				
Total				
Average (divide by 10)				
Implementation, Training, and Technical Support				
Efficient use of practice time				
Good staff training				
Fee to train is reasonable				
Vendor pays for consultant to implement				
Reliable technical support				
User groups or forums available?				

continued

TABLE 3-8

Scorecard for Vendor Selection cont'd

Area of Interest	Vendor 1	Vendor 2	Vendor 3	Comments
	Scoring: 1 = low; 5 = high			
Total				
Average (divide by 5)				
Note: Your practice may wish to give added weight to one or more areas of interest				
Upgrades				
Who decides timing of upgrades (if fee for upgrade required by vendor, prefer practice decides timing)?				
Fee or cost to upgrade				
Are upgrades compatible with HL7's EHR functional descriptors? (See Chapter 6)				
How often are upgrades suggested or required?				
Total				
Average (divide by 4) *Note: Your practice may wish to give added weight to one or more areas of interest*				
Physician-Patient Communications				
Physician can communicate with patients electronically: secure e-mail, virtual office visits, telemedicine				
Appears easy for patients to use				
Patient data in medical record are accessible by patient				

continued

TABLE 3-8

Scorecard for Vendor Selection cont'd

Area of Interest	Vendor 1	Vendor 2	Vendor 3	Comments
	Scoring: 1 = low; 5 = high			
Patients will like ability to communicate directly with physician				
Patient's data merged into chart				
Ease of response to patients				
Total				
Average (divide by 5 Note: Your practice may wish to give added weight to one or more areas of interest)				
Certification				
Vendor has been certified by Certification Commission for Healthcare Information Technology (CCHIT) (the American Health Information Management Association [AHIMA], the Healthcare Information and Management Systems Society [HIMSS], and the National Alliance for Health Information Technology are founding members of CCHIT)				
Vendor's Market Presence				
Has been around for many years				
Likely to stay in business				
Likely to be fair in negotiating				
Would feel good referring the company				

continued

TABLE 3-8

Scorecard for Vendor Selection cont'd

Area of Interest	Vendor 1	Vendor 2	Vendor 3	Comments
		Scoring: 1 = low; 5 = high		
Total				
Average (divide by 4)				
Note: Your practice may wish to give added weight to one or more areas of interest				
Total All Averages				
Total of Averages				
Divide by 6				
OVERALL SCORE				

STEP 8: SCHEDULE ONSITE DEMONSTRATIONS

Most top EMR vendors will provide you with an online product demonstration—a good starting point, but it may not be enough information to make a purchase decision. The sales team is well trained to show the EMR's strengths in a road-show format. But you'll be using it for a host of problem-solving decisions, and it's the EMR's problem-solving capabilities that separate the sales team from the practicing physician's team.

At least two or three practice workforce members should participate in the demonstration. Ask if you can enter data during the demonstration. Then, enter data related to a somewhat complicated problem you recently solved or are currently working through, and evaluate the data you get from the software. You're not challenging the salesperson's knowledge, but you do want to challenge the software's capabilities. You may want to invite your IT consultant who regularly advises your practice on system issues to participate in the live demonstration. Some practices like to schedule a "shoot out" where two or three vendors conduct a 45-minute, back-to-back demonstration. Following is a list of questions that will help you learn more about an EMR during a demonstration.

Vendor Presence in the Marketplace

You want to determine how well the vendor knows your business and the level of trust the vendor has established in the marketplace. You also want to determine if the vendor will be around two years from now to update your software for new standards or to provide upgrades. Ask the following questions:

- What's the average size of practice that purchases your EMR?
- How many concurrent user licenses have you sold
  — For all practices?
  — For practices of my size?
  — For practices of my type?
- How much of your budget is spent on new-product development?
- How many technical support people do you have?
- What were your revenues last year? What do you think they will be this year?
- How well do you work with IT Consultants?
- Have you participated in any mergers or acquisitions?
- Ask for a copy of the vendor's financial statement, especially balance sheet, and request an opinion from the practice's accountant about the vendor's financial reliability.

Vendor EHR Certification

When David J. Brailer, MD, PhD, national coordinator for health information technology, rolled out the *Framework for Strategic Action Progress Report* on July 21, 2004, one element of the framework for health information technology adoption included a process for vendor certification.

Anyone with a computer can develop an EHR. You want to know whether the vendor measured its software against industry standards of performance as part of a rigorous evaluation and you want to know the results of that evaluation. According to Dr Brailer's office, the certification process will be monitored by the Certification Commission for Healthcare Information Technology (CCHIT). The American Health Information Management Association (AHIMA), the Healthcare Information and Management Systems Society (HIMSS), and the National Alliance for Healthcare Information Technology are founding members of CCHIT.

EHR Certification to Boost Physician Confidence

Interoperability is the name of the game as physicians and patients begin exchanging health information in real time. As quickly as a physician can download lab results onto a handheld PC, the physician can then choose to electronically or verbally communicate details of test results and treatment plans to the patient.

The Certification Commission for Healthcare Information Technology (CCHIT) wants to be sure the message between products used by physician and patient is compatible. Additional outcomes of certification should

- Reduce the risk of IT investment,
- Improve the functioning of the IT marketplace, and
- Facilitate IT adoption incentives by payers and purchasers.

No Fear EHR

"Most of the current EHR marketplace will likely be certified," said Mark Leavitt, MD, PhD, Commission Chair and Medical Director for Health Information Management Systems Society (HIMSS). "Certification is not meant to freeze the EHR market. Rather, it helps the physician who is not sure which EHR to purchase, by preventing interoperability dead-ends."

Dr. Leavitt explains that the secret sauce for physicians comes as payers prepare to offer financial incentives for EHR adoption. Insurers want more data on quality, and EHRs capture and report that kind of data. "Certification assures that this data interface between physicians and payers can work."

Your Role in Certification

According to Dr Leavitt, the Certification Commission plans to start identifying certification elements by taking inventory of available EHR standards. One set of standards, developed by HL7, is currently in draft standard for trial use stage. You can preview those standards online at www.hl7.org. Select Resources, then Select HL7 Standards and/or HL7 DSTU Comments.

Will Interoperability in Healthcare Work?

If you're using a laptop, it's possible that there's a Pentium chip inside your Dell Computer that operates in a Microsoft environment while a Motorola wireless card picks up data from one of a hundred wireless networks. All you know is that whether you're at the office, at the airport, or at your son's soccer game, you're connected.

Interoperability works when you use your ATM at another bank; it works when a Nextel customer calls a Cingular customer; or when you make phone calls, download email or order a birthday cake from your Blackberry. Now, it's healthcare's turn to thrive.

The commission, made up of key healthcare stakeholders, indicated the first-step of the certification process should be ready for pilot implementation by the summer of 2005. Second- and third-step certifications will be more thorough and follow in subsequent years.

Article reprinted with permission from the September/October 2004 issue of Physician's e-Health Report.[6]

Vendor Customer Service and Technical Support History

Customer service implementation strategy and technical support are vital to the success of your EHR system. Technical support must be present. "Your business senses should throw up a red flag when you hear the words, 'We're working on it. We'll have it done in a couple of months,'" says Will McHenry, president and CEO of Healthcare Counsel and founder of Physician's Support Group, Inc, a management service organization (MSO) servicing physicians throughout the Southeast.

"It's okay for a vendor to turn a problem over to the research and development departments, but you should not get the runaround when you need answers to your technical questions." Questions that you need to ask are:

- What do customers say about your EHR?
- What levels of customer service do you provide? (If you think you'll spend more than $10,000 a year on a vendor, that vendor should send someone to your practice. Period. Find out whether customer service is provided by telephone or if a technical person is available to come to your practice.)
- How long does it usually take between a call for technical support and actual response?
- Is tech support available 24/7?
- Do you charge a fee for technical support? (Some vendors provide 10 to 12 hours of initial training to admin staff and unlimited year-round support to physicians. Others provide support to anyone, but it is billed at different rates.)

Vendor System Interoperability and Integration

Any time your practice connects two or more software applications, the technical support team must ensure that the two systems are integrated. Integration means that the computers can talk to each other. Interoperability means that once both systems are integrated, you can open, read, and transmit images or data. Compare integration and interoperability to making a phone call.

A Sprint customer can call a Cingular customer because the systems are integrated and the integrated lines allow customers to communicate with each other. But a Sprint customer may not be able to open a digital photo sent by a Cingular customer unless both systems are interoperable.

Ask the following questions about integration and interoperability.

- Will your software *integrate* with my practice management system? My billing system?
- Will I be able to receive images from the lab? From the hospital? From patients? From specialists? (Is your software *interoperable* with systems used by other providers, such as specialists to whom I frequently refer my patients?)
- Is my computer hardware sufficient for your software to work efficiently? What will it cost to upgrade?
- Will your software work on my PDA, tablet PC, desktop, wireless computers, and so forth?

Vendor Implementation Plan

A typical EHR system may take 18 to 36 months to implement, depending on budget, technical preparedness, size of practice, and workforce acceptance. Become familiar with how the vendor will conduct implementation to ensure that physicians use the system once it's live. Ask the following questions:

- How much can I implement now, and what can I put off until later?
- If I implement one module now, what should it be? Keep in mind that e-prescribing will be a hot issue with Medicare by 2006, and you should consider implementing modules that help you conduct e-prescribing in the early phases of implementation.

Vendor Training Plan

Training is critical to adoption. A superior product is little more than a boat anchor if no one in the practice knows how to make the most of the EHR system. On the other hand, good training will immediately result in helping you lower your administrative costs. Questions to ask include:

- What is your training plan for our workforce members and the physician/clinical team?
- Do you have an ongoing training plan?
- What is your plan for training new workforce members?

Vendor Upgrade Plan

Electronic medical records and EHRs are still being refined, so evaluate vendors' methodologies for upgrades. Any vendor worth its salt is a member of the HL7 Standards Committee and is tracking implementation of the EHR Draft Standards for Trial Use (DSTU) addressed in Chapter 6. Vendors featured in this book are some of the more than 200 active members of the HL7 workgroup.

Some vendors automatically issue upgrades and then send you an invoice for the new software. Before you sign a contract, be clear about who determines when you'll need an upgrade, including whether it's free or for a fee.

STEP 9: ASK ABOUT THE RETURN ON INVESTMENT

Electronic medical records have been around long enough that every reputable vendor can show a return on investment (ROI). The key is how long it will take to achieve your ROI, especially if implementation takes a year or two. What modules will help you quickly recover your financial investment and what modules are good for long-term ROI? Does the ROI involve reduction of staff?

"Part of the ROI for a small physician practice is determining whether the EMR is better than buying a box of file folders and paying a medical records clerk $15 an hour to pull charts," said practice manager Will McHenry. "Will the EMR be more efficient than the $25,000 the physician pays the clerk year after year?"

Some initial investment can be recouped from a robust billing and coding system, he says. "Docs tend to undercode, rather than face charges of upcoding," he added. "An EMR that manages several functions not only eliminates paper charts, but also catches undercoding and advises physicians whether the visit was a two-, a three-, or a four-level visit."

Getting the patient involved in using the EMR/EHR also contributes to the ROI. Too often patients walk out of the office without making their co-pays, making it difficult and costly to collect. "Ask the patient to make the co-pay at the point of registration before seeing the physician," McHenry said. "Even better if that's done online during check-in."

STEP 10: NEGOTIATE THE CONTRACT

"Every contract has sections that are worth negotiating," McHenry said. With demand for EMRs as great as they are, it's no wonder a new community of EMR consultants is emerging, helping physicians evaluate and make decisions on which EMR/EHR system is right for the practice specialty, staffing and technology requirements, and budget.

"Since EMRs, like cars, come with different sets of features, buyers should use this leverage to negotiate a good deal," wrote the authors of the Forrester Research Report, *Electronic Medical Records: A Buyer's Guide for Small Physician Practices.* "Electronic interfaces connect EMRs to testing labs but usually at added expense. Alerts don't fire off until data parameters get entered into the system. Disease-specific templates and guidelines, scheduling modules, and prescription management tools typically cost more. Given the competition for customers, it should be possible to get some of these bells and whistles at no extra charge."[2]

Other areas worth negotiating include:

- **Ownership of data, especially in an ASP-based model.** Many contracts indicate that the physician's practice owns the data. But if you cancel the EMR contract, you want to be sure the data that the EMR vendor holds in storage are readable, functional, and transferable to another system. If it's encrypted, you want it decrypted, and you'll want your data returned to you in a workable file that can be easily downloaded into another system. *Make sure that*

  - *The data ownership provision is spelled out clearly in the contract.*

  - *Any data conversion costs at the end of the contract are reasonable and specified in the contract.*

  - *Your attorney reviews the language before signing the contract.*

- **Additional training and technical support.** Training must be included for new and reassigned workforce members, especially since turnover can be a significant problem for physician practices.

- **Fee-based upgrades.** Who determines when you need upgrades? The practice or the vendor? About half the vendors we interviewed do not charge for monthly or quarterly upgrades, but they may charge a small fee for annual upgrades or version changes. Find out how disruptive any such change will be to your workflow.

- **Unlimited training and technical support for the physician.** Physicians often analyze charts and data after hours, so give extra consideration to a vendor with 24-hour technical support.

- **Co-op purchasing with several practices to share the costs and get a group rate**. Winona Health's case study that follows is an excellent example of a health community coming together to share costs and implementation of an EHR system.

- **Purchasing the hardware outright and negotiating only the price of the software.** You can eliminate the EHR vendor's markup (which is usually 4 to 5%) by learning the software system's requirements and purchasing hardware directly from the manufacturer.

Case Study: How We Share EMR Costs

Bill Davis, MD
Chief Medical Information Officer of Winona Health and Chief Financial
Officer and partner in Family Medicine of Winona, PA
Winona, Minnesota

When we needed an EMR, our healthcare community went together to make the purchase. It made us more efficient, and we all shared the cost of a common EMR. In a small city, the purchase collaboration is what made our EMR opportunity work.

Winona, Minnesota, is a small city with a big heart, nestled between the bluffs and the mighty Mississippi River. It is surrounded by spectacular natural beauty, wrapped in history, and steeped in cultural legacy. From a healthcare perspective, it lives in the shadow of Mayo Clinic and a 450 multi-specialty physician network 40 miles from Winona.

Our people here prefer the small town, friendly environment and they want their healthcare to be compatible with their lifestyle. In 1994, the community created Winona Health, an "umbrella" nonprofit organization for our residents. The organization consists of provider collaborators: the Winona Clinic (a multi-specialty group), Winona Family Medicine, and Winona Health, a regional health system. Today, our facilities range from Community Memorial Hospital's Family Birth Center and primary care hospital, primary care and multi-specialty physician clinics, assisted living communities, skilled nursing home, home care and hospice services.

When we decided to go to an EMR environment, we were convinced that it had to be a single shared record that could be accessed by Winona's residents as well as providers. Cerner's IQHealth selected us to be an alpha site to test and develop a patient portal record. Winona's Community Memorial Hospital is the general contractor for the EMR, but the physicians share in the cost, which makes the EMR much more affordable for everyone.

Now that we're live as a full client, our cost is about $5,000 per year per physician.

Existing patients of Winona Health can access their Personal Medical Record online at home, from kiosks at Community Hospital, the pharmacy, the local mall, or other public places.

The biggest improvement has been in patient safety because the portal provides us with automatic drug interactions and allergies. A couple of times a day, I still remind patients of allergies because they forget.

Physicians can also query for potential problems. I might not remember if a patient is on blood thinners, but the EMR reminds me of a bleeding episode at the hospital several months back. I can send a prescription online to the pharmacy in our network, and I can download a template that contains medical details for a single health issue such as bronchitis. I usually customize each record from the template, but by noon, I'm done logging details from my morning patients. And, by the end of the day I've finished transcribing details from

continued

all my patients. In the process, I've eliminated nearly $20,000 a year in dictation costs.

I've used computers that have made my life worse for me, but now that EMRs are searchable and much more doctor-friendly, I'm very comfortable looking at the patient chart in an electronic format. I'm just not flipping pages anymore, hoping I won't miss anything.

Reprinted with permission from the May/June 2004 issue of Physician's e-Health Report.[7] Dr. Davis can be reached at wdavis@winonafamilymedicine.org.

STEP 11: AGREE ON A PURCHASE PLAN

"Physicians tend to defer buying decisions if they don't see the immediate business advantage," says Will McHenry. "That's why it's important to discuss the purchase plan with a practice management consultant or accountant."

Most small physician practices don't have $25,000 to $100,000 lying around to invest in new software and may need financial advice. The amount and types of loans available to physician practices are usually governed by:

- Creditworthiness
- Length of time in the practice
- Time to retirement age
- Banking relationships

The software you select will dictate the type of financing arrangements you obtain. "If you're a small or solo practice, the monthly service fee for an ASP model will be more attractive and less likely to need a bank's involvement," McHenry said. "Users of ASP models don't have to pay off a large debt, don't have to worry about technology support or automatic updates because the software is housed offsite and maintained by the vendor." "Subscribing to an ASP model is usually less expensive if you plan to use it for three to five years," McHenry said. "And most ASP vendors will want you to sign a multiyear agreement. If it's for a longer period of time, then a subscription will be more expensive than a software license."

Remember to protect your data if you think you will move from one vendor to another.

In his article, "Financing High Tech: You Can Afford It After All," reporter Tyler Chin states[8]:

Generally, physicians can seek a lease-to-own arrangement or a straight loan from a lease company or a bank, or go with a subscription pricing model arrangement through the technology vendor.

Under the terms of a lease-to-own or bank-financing arrangement, the lender forks over the full purchase price to the seller. A doctor then must make monthly payments to the lender over an agreed-upon period, which typically ranges from three to five years. The lender owns the goods until the physician pays off the loan plus a dollar buyout payment, at which time the physician owns the goods.

Vendors often have relationships with leasing companies that likely provide a lease arrangement with any physician the vendor does business with. "Consult with both a lease company and a bank," McHenry said. "But go with the best interest rate and the financier that offers the best overall service."

STEP 12: ASK FOR HELP WHEN YOU NEED IT

In true entrepreneurial spirit, a new cottage industry has evolved to help physicians select and implement a new EMR. Your practice management consultant or EMR consultant are good resources to understand how your practice runs and should be able to help with EHR system selection.

Trust a health law or IT attorney to guide you through the contract.

You can hire a consultant to act as a buyer's agent for you, but first check that the buyer's agent is not under contract to represent only one or two EMR vendors. Expect your consultant to do some or all of the following:

- Interview your office manager to learn about your culture and workflow
- Work with the physician champions to learn what they want in an EMR
- Agree to evaluate vendors that fit your financial conditions and requirements
- Work with your implementation team to find EMR vendors that fit your business and culture
- Develop an implementation timetable
- Assist in negotiating a contract
- Assist in finding funding

Check the credentials of EMR consultants before hiring an agent to select an EMR for you.

INCLUDE THE PATIENT IN THE ELECTRONIC MEDICAL RECORDS/ELECTRONIC HEALTH RECORDS PROCUREMENT PROCESS

The EMR movement has languished for more than two decades. But now that EHRs are in the hands of policymakers, elected officials, advocate groups, and consumers, the movement will progress more quickly, not only in the United States but also around the world. Consumers in Europe,

Asia, Australia, and America understand the basics of how EHRs can be used. Healthcare consumers and employers are seeking strategies to reduce financial hardships from increased healthcare premiums and decreased benefits, medical errors, and poor disease management caused by what Newt Gingrich calls "archaic information systems of our hospitals and clinics that directly affect the quality of care we receive."[10]

Some Early-Adopter Consumer/Patients Already Own Personal Health Records

If the health system's infrastructure moves like clockwork, patient involvement, which has already begun, is expected to mature between 2006 and 2008, or as soon as standard formats become available and are in the hands of technology entrepreneurs.

One format for electronic health records discussed in Chapter 1 is personal health records (PHR). Before 2010, PHRs will become as common a term as ATMs. An ATM card helps consumers manage banking data, and a PHR helps consumers manage health information.

A PHR is controlled by the patient. Health information can be created by the patient, such as a daily health diary for patients treated for chronic diseases. Inside the medical office, the physician and patient can review the diary to learn more about the patient's condition and treatment options.

A PHR may also contain family histories of illness, emergency contact information, a living will or advance directive, allergies and adverse reactions, blood types, and so on.

With so much clinical and administrative information available to both patient and physician, it is in the best interest of physicians to teach patients how to use PHRs. Personal health records are especially helpful when registering a new patient to the practice.

The White House goal is to have PHRs used in e-prescribing before the end of the decade. It's going to be an exciting transformation.

How the Federal Government Plans to Help

For years, the Veterans Administration has implemented and refined its EMR software, servicing four million veterans a year at 128 sites with point-of-care data. The software, called VistA, is now available for free, due to the Freedom of Information Act. Through a grant from CMS, a VistA Office (formerly called VistA *Lite*) has been designed specifically for use in clinics and physicians offices.

CMS sent out a call on December 2, 2004, asking physicians to help test VistA Office. The ideal practice size is one to eight clinicians. A demo version of VistA is available at www.va.gov/vista.[11] To inquire about participation, consult the Iowa Foundation for Medical Care, (www.ifmc.org) or send an email to VistA@ifmc.org.

Market Institutions

Executive Order 13335 directed the Office of the National Coordinator for Health Information Technology (Dr. David Brailer is the first HIT coordinator) to develop, maintain, and direct the implementation of a strategic plan to guide the nation's implementation of interoperable health information technology (HIT) in both the public and private healthcare sectors. The national implementation plan, divided into three phases, begins by establishing "market institutions" to support clinicians as they procure and use IT. The presence of market institutions will help stabilize the market and create a better environment for investment and accountability, lower the risk of HIT procurement, and make more efficient use of your investment.

A relatively new organization, the Physicians EHR Coalition (PEHRC), is an example of a market institution. It is made up of 14 physician organizations with a goal to help small to midsize physician practices deploy electronic health records in their practices.

"While physicians are adopting information technology in growing numbers, there remain substantial economic and technical barriers to full-scale deployment of electronic health records, especially in small- and medium-size medical practices. PEHRC will allow physicians to address these barriers with a unified voice, and be powerful advocates for putting health information technology in the service of quality of care," said PEHRC co-chair David C. Kibbe, MD.[9]

SUMMARY

The actual implementation process is as much about culture management as it is about scheduling and training. That's why we've devoted the next chapter to help you plan and customize the actual transition to electronics in your practice.

ENDNOTES

1. Hagland M. Reality EMRs: coming soon to an organization near you—electronic record keeping. *Healthcare Informatics.* 2004;21:36.

2. Barrett MJ, Holmes BJ, McAulay S. *Electronic Medical Records: A Buyer's Guide for Small Physician Practice.* Oakland, Calif: California Health Care Foundation (prepared by Forrester Research); 2003:13.

3. Definition provided by the Healthcare Information and Management Systems Society (HIMSS). Available at: www.himss.org/ASP/ContentRedirector.asp?ContentId=54797.

4. Anderson MR. *Information Technology Trends and Solutions: 2004 Summary Report. Extensive Evaluation Ranks Top Electronic Medical Record Applications.*

Available at: www.acgroup.org. (The detailed 160+ page report is also available at that site for a fee. The summary report is reprinted with permission in Appendix C of this book.)

5. 15th Annual Health Information Management Systems Society Leadership Survey. (Sponsored by Superior Consultant Company.) Available at: www.himss.org/2004survey/ASP/index.asp.

6. EHR certification to boost physician confidence. *Physician's e-Health Report.* September–October 2004, Volume 1, Number 5.

7. Focus on physician column: how we share EMR costs. *Physician's e-Health Report.* May/June 2004. Available at: www.physiciansehr.com.

8. Chin T. Financing high-tech: you can afford it after all. *AMNews.* March 8, 2004.

9. Premier Medical Organizations Announce Formation of Physicians Electronic Health Record Coalition. News release, July 22, 2004. Available at: www.aafp.org/x28539.xml.

10. Gingrich N, Kennedy P. Operating in a vacuum. *The New York Times.* May 3, 2004.

11. Send an e-mail message to nanthracite@comcast.net for instructions about where to download the VistA demo for use on a Windows PC with a demo version of Caché from InterSystems. A version for use with Linux and GTM can be found on the WorldVistA site at http://sourceforge.net/projects/worldvista.

chapter 4

Making the Switch From Paper to Electronic Medical Records

In his article, "Training Is the Key," Robert Lowes, senior editor of *Medical Economics* magazine, compares the implementation process of an electronic medical record (EMR) to learning how to play a piano.[1] Some physicians will learn how to play Beethoven's *Moonlight Sonata* while others will end up playing *Chopsticks*. If you're looking for a sonata, first evaluate your workflow and then work with the EMR vendor to customize modules that work for you and your workforce. Finally, you must use the software until you have learned how to make it sing for you. Without knowing how your work flows, and without regular use, the vendor will implement modules that have worked in other practices, but not necessarily for yours. The result is likely to be choppy integration.

WHAT YOU WILL LEARN IN THIS CHAPTER

- How to switch from using paper to electronic records in 10 steps
- How to plan for training and implementation
- How to celebrate small victories

STEP 1: PLAN THE IMPLEMENTATION

If you've laid the groundwork by involving your workforce in the EMR selection, the implementation stage shouldn't be a huge surprise. Even so, everyone will come to "roll-out day" with a slightly different idea of how things were supposed to take place.

"In most cases, you can manage resistance by keeping people informed. People need to have a line of sight—they need to know what's in it for them. Express the positive, but tell the truth," said Doug Ens, President, EMR Institute (www.emrinstitute.com), an organization that helps physicians through the EMR selection and implementation process. Ens has helped more than 250 physician practices implement an EHR.

Ens said the types of resistance behavior practices are likely to experience include:

- Retaining old habits and failure to adapt to e-way
- Hoarding of knowledge that someone has about a process
- Apathy in training or staff meetings
- Sarcasm and public criticism of the tool

To counter this behavior, develop a systematic method to get suggestions for improvement or make recommendations for future releases of the product.

"Find a few staff members who tend to be influencers and empower them early on to serve as your technology champions," Ens said. "As resistance subsides, put others into power roles such as train the trainer, and enable them to teach others what they've learned."

Paul Peterson, sales and marketing manager for Allscripts Healthcare Solutions (www.allscripts.com), recommends adopting a hybrid EMR, one that is both paperless and paper-based. "Let your staff get used to doing one thing new," he said. "Adopt one module, like document entry or patient charting, so that everyone adjusts to the new way of processing information. Then, move into e-prescribing or online patient communications."

Until the EMR is interoperable, limit paper-based activities to:

- Lab reports
- Imaging
- Communications with other specialties and hospitals

Peterson cautions physicians to not fall into the trap of creating a duplicate medical chart. "Part of the process is determining who does what, for example, when a paper lab report is faxed to the office. You don't want the report sitting on the physician's desk if the hybrid EMR process requires someone to enter the data into the patient's chart," he said.

STEP 2: KNOW YOUR WORKFLOW

Map your workflow using flowcharts or the modified flowcharts from Chapter 2. Do not skip this process. Your workflow may not replicate those in Chapter 2 but they will be similar. Develop workflows on paper and deliver the charts to the software vendor you have selected for your practice. This process will help the vendor understand who needs training and on what functions.

STEP 3: TRANSITION PAPER TO ELECTRONICS AS PART OF YOUR ELECTRONIC MEDICAL RECORD IMPLEMENTATION WORKFLOW

We can all learn from the early adopters when moving from paper charts to an EMR. In the more than 50 telephone and in-person interviews we conducted with physicians while writing this book, we found several successful strategies.

- Every person in the office understood that the process of switching from a paper-based system to an EMR would take a long time.
- Most practices adopted a hybrid EMR for the first 6 to 18 months.
- Most practices implemented the EMR with more than one clinical team at a time, or implement the EMR practice-wide. Generally, the one physician-nurse clinical team in a group practice met with more resistance than if the teams could compare and support implementation success.

Physicians at the 2004 *Toward an Electronic Patient Record* (TEPR) conference said that during the implementation stage, they brought both electronic and paper records to the first three patient visits. Duplicate patient records is anathema to physicians, but try following these tactics to minimize the disruption:

- On the patient's first electronic visit, ask the patient to provide family medical history via an online visit to your Web site or through a kiosk at the office, if either is available.
- Gather critical information about the patient for the electronic record on the first medical visit. Critical information includes contact information, medical diagnosis, current medications, allergies, adverse reactions, and insurance information.
- The first week of information gathering is likely to be slower than usual, so lighten your patient load for the week you implement your EMR.
- By the patient's third visit, most of the patient record has been duplicated in the electronic record.

Physicians who use optical scanners to transfer paper to electronic records offered mixed reviews about the technology. If the scanning software is unable to convert images into data, such as through optical character recognition (OCR), then the patient record information may not be searchable. The practice, then, has little more than an electronic image taking up space on the computer. That may save on physical space in the practice devoted to paper records, but it does not provide the potential productivity of being able to access, analyze, and communicate salient characteristics of patients' records.

In transitioning to a paperless practice, a hybrid EMR comes with a few dos and don'ts, which are outlined in Table 4-1.

TABLE 4-1

Dos and Don'ts When Transitioning From Paper to Electronic Records

Hybrid EMR Dos	Hybrid EMR Don'ts
■ Set aside resources and time for training	■ Do the training or implementation yourself; lack of training is the biggest reason for failed EMRs
■ Reduce patient load for a week during implementation	■ Schedule implementation during peak flu or cold season
■ Watch for paper triggers; compare what you designed to be workflow to what actually happens	■ Create "shadow" or duplicate records
■ Expect meltdowns for the first week; these will subside within 2 months	■ Expect your vendor to be present for training and technical support
■ Build new patient records electronically	■ Assume scanned documents are searchable; "techies" call scanned documents "dumb documents," which require conversion, balancing, and validation to be searchable
■ Expect the practice's champion to step up and offer encouragement, even when you make mistakes	
■ Provide a refresher course on HIPAA Privacy and Security Rules policies and procedures	■ Permit punitive actions during the learning cycle
■ Expect the vendor to accommodate your specialty's needs	■ Implement a Web site or EMR capabilities without HIPAA privacy and security measures in place
■ Train your patients on how to securely access and use the EMR; ask if your patients will provide you with their e-mail addresses	■ Do this alone; keep your vendors or IT consultants involved
	■ Leave patients out of the adoption equation
■ Expect continued progress and IT adoption from your healthcare partners	■ Expect miracles; do expect collaboration

EMR indicates electronic medical record; HIPAA, Health Insurance Portability and Accountability Act of 1996; IT, information technology.

STEP 4: CREATE A COMBINATION OF TRAINING EXPERIENCES FOR YOUR WORKFORCE

People learn in a variety of ways. For example, healthcare professionals tend to be visual learners rather than auditory learners, so be sure your vendor or consultant includes plenty of visual or hands-on opportunities for you and your workforce. Some of the more popular training experiences follow.

■ **Webinars:** Most vendors have developed very effective video training seminars offered on the Web, or "Webinars." These are particularly helpful when training needs to be presented to many employees with varying schedules, or when your workforce needs a refresher.

Webinars work well as an independent learning tool, particularly in midsize to large practices. Ask the vendor to provide your workforce with unlimited access so that each member can access a training module, similar to a help desk or tutorial. However, an online course should not take the place of other training media, such as quick reference guides and in-person training.

- **Printed Quick Reference Guides:** Most users are familiar with quick reference guides that include screen shots accompanied by simple instructions on how to successfully enter data on the screen.

- **In-person Training:** Nothing takes the place of human interaction when a problem exists between the keyboard and the person using the system. Also, be sure to bring refreshments to the in-person training sessions.

- **Online Help Desk or Technical Support:** Information moves quickly in a physician's practice, and a good EMR vendor will provide 24-hour technical support.

- **In-house Coaching:** By far, EHR-trained staff provides the most immediate training response. Even so, a vendor or EHR consultant must stay in contact for updates and troubleshooting.

STEP 5: PROVIDE COMPUTER TRAINING TO THE "E-CHALLENGED"

People who don't know about computers may be threatened or fear they'll touch something that will destroy data. Minimize that fear by teaching the basics of how to use personal computers, Microsoft® Windows®, and e-mail features. Choose a member of the practice workforce who can "hand hold" those who are adapting to electronic workflows and processes in the practice. Or, select software that can be downloaded to a tablet PC so that the e-challenged can access information with a stylus.

STEP 6: PREPARE YOUR WORKFORCE BY USING KEY MESSAGES

Your workforce members are most likely to accept EMR training if (1) they do not believe their jobs are threatened if they don't adapt to the technology right away; and (2) they believe everyone is essentially learning new processes for managing information in the practice. Examples of key messages include:

- We're going to learn how to do this together
- This is as new to me as it is to you
- There will be changes in how we manage our work, but I think you'll like those changes

- We're looking for coaches and teams to work together on this
- The technology isn't perfect yet, so if your team finds something that isn't working, let one of your team members know
- We welcome your suggestions on how to make the practice's information management processes better

STEP 7: GIVE CONTENT TIME TO SINK IN

On the day your workforce will be involved with in-person training, cut back your patient schedule to avoid distractions. This will improve concentration and make the most of your training investment.

Learn one or two modules at a time. A 12-day session for Misys Healthcare Systems (www.misyshealthcare.com) customers is really several 2- to 3-day chunks spread out over six to nine months. This gives the workforce time to build knowledge of one module before moving on to the next.

STEP 8: DEVELOP INTERNAL TRAINERS

Internal trainers are workforce members who are coaches to peers and supervisors as well as trainers to new employees. Internal trainers are non-judgmental, supportive, and personable. They know how your work flows, and they should be trained to help other workforce members understand how the software is best used for your purposes.

STEP 9: MAKE A PRACTICE-WIDE COMMITMENT TO ENTER CLINICAL DATA

Of the more than 50 physicians we interviewed for this book, all of them said that if there hadn't been at least one physician champion in each of their practices, EMR adoption would likely have failed. Everyone in the office—including the physicians—must commit to the change.

"It's like learning to play an instrument or learning how to use the Internet," Doug Holmes, MD, said about implementing the Misys Healthcare Systems EMR. "It's slow at first and people make mistakes. But it gets faster. Once you learn how to use it, you'll never go back to paper," he said.

Pediatrician and practice manager Jerry Bernstein, MD, went live with an EMR from A4 Health Systems (www.a4healthsystems.com) in 1 week. "After discussing the switch to electronic medical records (EMR) with my colleagues, our practice made the decision to go 'cold turkey' to electronic medical records," Bernstein said. "We all had our meltdowns during the first days, but I was surprised at how quickly the clinical staff learned how to use an electronic system."

As part of the implementation plan, the practice scheduled fewer patients during the go-live week and made sure the vendor's tech people were on site at both offices. Now, each physician carries a small laptop into each examining room and downloads patient records stored on the in-house server. With the wireless network, the physicians can also readily access the Internet on the spot for medical information, if needed.

"Our EMR doesn't help us see patients more quickly. But it does allow much more efficiency, more accuracy, and more accountability. Costs saved from outsourcing to transcription companies allowed us to experience a return on investment within six months. We didn't lose anyone on staff; instead, we shifted and retrained," Bernstein said.

STEP 10: CELEBRATE SMALL VICTORIES

The move to EMRs is a culture change. Change brings resistance and joy. Acknowledge the small things so that everyone in the practice finds satisfaction. For example, here are a few of the "small things" you can do to help ease the transition:

■ Give recognition to both the mentor (coach) and protégé when a significant problem is solved

■ If EMR training is presented after hours, pay your workforce for attending

■ Reward employees for sharing computer techniques and tips

■ Have a party when you exceed pre-EMR productivity

THE NEXT STEPS: INTEGRATION AND INTEROPERABILITY

Congratulations! If you've followed the implementation steps outlined in this chapter, you've made significant strides that will bring your practice into the 21st century. Now, you're ready to take your implementation program outside the practice by following some principles of computer science.

The easiest method to integrate software from multiple provider sources is to have everyone in your provider community using the same tablet PCs and software (for PDAs, document archiving, practice management, speech recognition, and so on). The alternative is to agree on standards that make clinical data interoperable.

If you read our book, *HIPAA Transactions: A Nontechnical Business Guide for Healthcare* (AMA Press; 2004), you learned that your billing and coding services vendors, working with your in-house (or contracted) coders, are exchanging HIPAA-compliant transactions to public and private payers. The Centers for Medicare and Medicaid Services (CMS) requires that if you are in a practice of 10 or more full-time equivalents, you must submit HIPAA-compliant transactions or CMS will delay reimbursement for services for an additional 14 days. (A *HIPAA-compliant* transaction means that you have met administrative, physical, and technical requirements in HIPAA's Privacy and Security Rules and that your billing company can exchange billing and coding information through the payment system and make direct deposits into your account.)

When it comes to EHR integration and interoperability, you will be performing a similar exchange of data, but in an EHR system, the exchange contains clinical information about your patients. Clinical data is of high value to your practice and for privacy, security, and financial reasons, must be closely guarded. Just as with billing and coding data flow, clinical data must meet specific standards so that labs, hospitals, specialists, payers, and so on, can access the portions that are accessible to them and respond with data that is important to your patient's care. Part II of this book addresses how the Health Level Seven (HL7) standards are being tested, and where you can have input on their development and approval.

Begin Interoperability With One Module

You've come a long way in your EHR implementation, and to experience real value for your practice and patients, it's appropriate to want to focus on the electronic sharing of files, especially with labs, hospitals, specialists, and pharmacies. The healthcare industry doesn't yet have all of the answers on how to make clinical data interoperable in a national or international setting.[2] But we do know that information technology protocols are in place for you to conduct several clinical transactions. Nearly all EHR vendors currently communicate using the XML programming language. Capabilities for you to exchange electronic files with pharmacies have been in place for more than five years.

Let's say you want to start with e-prescribing, which includes e-faxing and making wireless transmissions. Once you've selected your e-prescribing software vendor, your vendor and/or implementation consultant can help you set up that connectivity and staff training. Follow these steps to test data exchanges between your practice and the pharmacy.

1.   Ensure your HIPAA Privacy and Security procedures are in place.
2.   Identify two or three pharmacies that you use most frequently and ask if they can accept wireless or e-fax transactions from you. Your software vendor or consultant should share computer formatting language with the pharmacy. The National Council for Prescription Drug Programs (NCPDP) script is recommended as a foundational standard for e-prescribing messages. Until you apply for, and are assigned your national provider identifier (NPI), use your NCPDP provider identifier.
3.   With your vendor's help, develop a fictitious patient file, using one of your most commonly prescribed medications. Some vendors have

fictitious patient files already in place, but we recommend you do set up a file with the vendor's guidance.

4. Determine whether you need prior authorizations between prescribers and payers before sending the prescription. (Is the prescription in the specific payer's formulary?)

5. Submit the test file to the pharmacy's pilot test site. You should receive a response that lets you know whether the prescription was accepted; and if not, the response will provide a reason why the transaction was not completed.

6. If you are using an EHR to electronically send the prescription, verify that the prescription was also logged into the fictitious patient's medical record.

Continuity of Care Record Harmonizes With EHRs

On November 7, 2004, HL7 and ASTM International[3] demonstrated that ASTM's Continuity of Care Record (CCR) can be implemented as an HL7 Version 3 (V3) Clinical Document Architecture XML document.

According to the Center for Health Information Technology (CHiT) (www.centerforhit.org),

> the CCR is being developed in response to the need to organize and make transportable a set of basic information about a patient's health care that is accessible to clinicians and patients. It is intended to foster and improve continuity of care, reduce medical errors, and ensure a minimum standard of secure health information transportability. Adoption of the CCR by the medical community and IT vendors will be a first step in achieving interoperability of medical records.
>
> The CCR will be a digital file, producible using readily available software such as Microsoft® Word, or generated from hospital or practice EHR systems. Because the CCR will be a simple XML document, different EHR systems will be able to exchange—import and export—the CCR. In addition, because the CCR data will be in XML it can be displayed in a variety of formats, such as HL7 messages, HTML (browser), PDFs, and Word.

The CCR is being developed by the American Academy of Family Physicians, the Massachusetts Medical Society, the American Medical Association, the American Academy of Pediatrics, the Health Information Management and Systems Society, and the American Health Care Association, with the standards-development organization ASTM International.

SUMMARY

You are in good company if you are making the transition from paper to EMRs. You don't have to be a technical wizard, but your implementation team must include one person who understands how work flows in the practice, and you must have at least one physician who will champion the move to EMRs. Don't expect everyone to be thrilled about the transition, but do expect everyone to make an effort to learn—and regularly use—the new method of managing health information.

In Part 1 of this book, we provided an overview of where we are in health information technology, and where we are headed. We showed you how to map out your workflow so that you can select a vendor that is a good fit for your practice specialty and culture. We showed you how to evaluate and select a vendor, how to move from a paper-based to an electronic environment, and how to blend training experiences for your workforce. This chapter concludes the practical side of EMR evaluation, selection, transition, and implementation.

In Part 2 we present the results of new federal initiatives in the clinical sector of healthcare (Chapter 5) and present the electronic health record (EHR) standards in test stage—what they will mean and how you would use them if they become the final standard in 2006 (Chapter 6).

ENDNOTES

1. Lowes R. EMR success: training is the key. *Med Econ.* 2004;81:11. Available at: www.providersedge.com/ehdocs/ehr_articles/EMR_Success-Training_is_the_Key.pdf.

2. Electronic integration and interoperability are focus areas for several association workgroup sessions, including the Office of the National Coordinator for Health Information Technology (ONCHIT), Physicians Electronic Health Record Coalition (PEHRC), URAC, Regional Health Information Organizations (RHIOs), the Workgroup for Electronic Data Interchange (WEDI), American Health Information Management Association (AHIMA), and Health Information Management Systems Society (HIMSS).

3. ASTM International, originally known as the American Society for Testing and Materials (ASTM), was formed over a century ago, when engineers and scientists got together to address frequent rail breaks in the burgeoning railroad industry. Their work led to standardization on the steel used in rail construction, ultimately improving railroad safety for the public. Today, ASTM continues to be the standards forum of choice of a diverse range of industries that come together under the ASTM umbrella to solve standardization challenges.

PART 2

Standards Relevant to the Physician's Practice

chapter 5

Clinical Data Set Standards for Providers

*In theory, there is no difference between theory and practice.
In practice there is.*—**Yogi Berra**[1]

Chapters 5 and 6 discuss the results of new federal initiatives in the clinical sector of healthcare. This chapter focuses on the background of those federal initiatives and outlines the standards adopted for the federal system under the Consolidated Health Informatics program.

WHAT YOU WILL LEARN IN THIS CHAPTER

■ Why the federal government has taken a new approach to technology in the clinical sector of the healthcare industry
■ What the Consolidated Health Informatics program covers
■ The role of standards organizations in developing these programs
■ The role of the Health Insurance Portability and Accountability Act of 1996 (HIPAA) Administrative Simplification standards with regard to these new initiatives
■ What data element code sets are included in the clinical initiatives

Key Terms

Clinical Vocabularies: Standard code sets that will be understood by practitioners who have access to the "dictionary" of terms and uses.

continued

Consolidated Health Informatics (CHI): A federal initiative that requires federal agencies that engage in healthcare activities to adopt a common set of clinical, administrative, and messaging standards.

Messaging Standards: The protocols for transmitting information between sender and receiver, whereby the receiver understands what the sender intended to convey.

THE GOVERNMENT'S APPROACH TO ELECTRONIC MEDICAL RECORDS AND ELECTRONIC HEALTH RECORDS

Earlier in this book, we discussed the characteristics of electronic medical records (EMRs) and the practical steps that will help you select, purchase, and implement EMRs. If you are evaluating EMRs for your practice, you may have found that there are considerable differences in how current EMRs function. The theory being evaluated by several associations and government agencies is that these variations may be minimized by standardizing functions, data elements, and communication protocols. These standards would help the healthcare industry achieve key objectives of using EMRs. .

In the past two years, there has been a fundamental shift by the federal government in how it implements healthcare policy, especially as it relates to adoption of electronic processes. Previously, the federal government's attention was focused on *administrative processes*, using the authority of Administrative Simplification provisions of the Health Insurance Portability and Accountability Act of 1996 (HIPAA) and the Administrative Procedures Act to make rules for transactions and code sets, privacy, security, and identifiers.[2] Although the federal government continues to implement the Administrative Simplification standards under the Administrative Procedures Act, it also is implementing electronic *clinical* functions, data elements, messaging, and process standards using a different approach.

In December 2002, the Bush Administration began implementing the *E-Gov* initiative, following enactment of HR 2458, the E-Government Act of 2002.[3] The Consolidated Health Informatics (CHI) program is part of that initiative. In July 2003, US Department of Health and Human Services (HHS) Secretary Tommy Thompson announced two initiatives designed for "building a national electronic healthcare system that will allow patients and their doctors to assess their complete medical records anytime and anywhere they are needed. . . ."[4]

1. In May 2004, Secretary Thompson announced the appointment of a National Health Information Technology Coordinator to coordinate and accelerate US "health information technology efforts."[5]

2. In July 2004, Secretary Thompson initiated "a 10-year plan to build a national electronic health information infrastructure in the United States" and outlined "four major collaborative goals" and "12 strategies for advancing and focusing future efforts."[6] (The plan, goals, and strategies are discussed in Chapter 6, along with prospective *functional descriptor* standards pertaining to EHRs two-year testing of which began in July 2004,[7] following Health Level Seven [HL7] ballot approval announced by Secretary Thompson in May 2004).[5]

This chapter focuses on the CHI initiative, which is being adopted by all federal agencies that engage in healthcare activities.

FEDERAL GOVERNMENT'S E-GOVERNMENT PROGRAM

The term *E-Government*, or *E-Gov*, simply means electronic government. The Bush Administration outlined this initiative in its February 2002 budget message to Congress, stressing the need for the federal government to be "more focused on citizens and results," using "improved Internet-based technology to make it easy for citizens and businesses to interact with the government, save taxpayer dollars, and streamline citizen-to-government communications."[8] Within the E-Gov structure, the program includes "government-wide initiatives to integrate agency operations and information technology investments. The goal of these initiatives will be to eliminate redundant systems and significantly improve the government's quality of customer service for citizens and businesses."[8] The principles embodied in the budget message provided the foundation for HR 2458, the E-Government Act of 2002, which President Bush signed into law on December 17, 2002.[9]

On the E-Gov Web site (www.whitehouse.gov/omb/egov/site_map.htm), specific Presidential program initiatives are allocated to one of five separate E-Gov portfolios:

- Government to Citizen
- Government to Government
- Government to Business
- Internal Efficiency and Effectiveness
- E-Authentication

Within the Government to Business portfolio is the CHI initiative. Why is an initiative that focuses on standardizing management of healthcare information exchange and management in the federal government of interest to physicians in private practice?

First, federal programs comprise a significant market share in the healthcare industry, and federal programs such as Medicare play an important and growing role in private sector healthcare activities. As a result, the federal government's adoption of clinical standards through its employees and dependants, military branches, and Veterans Affairs hospitals will induce the private sector to adopt the same standards. The inducement is accompanied by incentives, such as licensing by the federal government of clinical vocabularies such as Systematized Nomenclature of Medicine-Clinical Terms (SNOMED-CT) and making it available to all US providers at no cost.

What's in a Name? Perhaps the Future of IT

By Joseph Goedert, News Editor, Health Data Management

December 2002—If a laboratory technician calls an "electrolyte panel" test a "Chem 4," a nurse calls it a "chemistry profile," and a physician refers to it simply as "electrolytes," will an electronic medical records system know that all three references mean the same thing? If there is no standardization of clinical vocabularies in patient records, how can provider organizations efficiently gather and analyze clinical data to assess the quality of care?

The answer, says Matthew Morgan, MD, is that they can't.

"Physicians speak in a combination of natural language and acronyms," says Morgan, a practicing general internist and director of healthcare informatics at Per-Se Technologies Inc., Atlanta. "We have armies of people trying to decipher what physicians are doing when they treat patients." Morgan practices at University Health Network, a three-hospital academic system in Toronto.

In the past year, though, a number of factors have made standard clinical vocabularies move up the list of medical data priorities, industry experts say. These include:

- An industrywide consensus that clinical information systems must support patient safety initiatives as well as data collection and analysis.
- The marriage of two massive clinical vocabularies to form SNOMED Clinical Terminology, or SNOMED CT.
- The possibility of government-mandated standards for clinical vocabularies.

Consequently, interest in clinical vocabularies from clinical software vendors has grown. In the past year, 46 "major" healthcare information technology vendors along with many "niche" vendors have licensed SNOMED CT, says Diane Aschman, COO at SNOMED International, Northfield, Ill.

Article reprinted with permission from Health Data Management.[10]

Second, most private sector physicians are not isolated from federal healthcare activities, again with Medicare contributing a significant percentage of reimbursement for most physicians and hospitals and, possibly in the future, providing a relatively higher level of reimbursement for providers who adopt and use the clinical standards. Finally, as we shall see, clinical standards are adopted much faster and more efficiently than the regulatory process underpinning administrative standards covered under HIPAA. Table 5-1 outlines the CHI initiative, drawing on and reproducing information from the E-Gov Web site under the header "E-Gov at a Glance."[11]

TABLE 5-1

Attributes of the Consolidated Health Informatics Initiative

Description	Adopts a portfolio of existing health information interoperability standards (health vocabulary and messaging) enabling all agencies in the federal health enterprise to "speak the same language" based on common enterprise-wide business and information technology (IT) architectures.
Progress to Date	■ Government-wide health IT governance council established.
	■ Portfolio of 24 target domains for data and messaging standards identified.
	■ Four messaging and one health vocabulary standards adopted government-wide; recommendations under review for remaining 19 clinical domains.[5] [*Authors' Note: Secretary Thompson announced adoption of 15 of these 19 clinical domains on May 6, 2004.*]
	■ Partnered with 23 federal agencies/departments that use health data for agreement to build adopted standards into their health IT architecture.
	■ Regular meetings with industry to prevent major incompatibilities in partnership with the National Committee on Vital and Health Statistics (NCVHS).
Next Steps	■ Facilitate implementation of adopted standards.
	■ Maintain adopted standards by working with standard development organizations.
	■ Continue adoption of new standards as needed to support Federal Health Architecture (FHA) line of business.
	■ Assess government-wide investments in standards' licenses and support.[12]
	■ Define change management role for the initiative.
	■ Provide requirements government-wide for health IT architecture standards.
	■ Identify appropriate pilots, demonstrations, and deployments.
	■ Incorporate Consolidated Health Informatics (CHI) goals into the FHA.

Source: White House Web site at: www.whitehouse.gov/omb/egov/downloads/e-gov_initiatives.htm. Accessed December 5, 2004.

Three important points can be drawn from Table 5-1:

- CHI only impacts *directly* federal government health-related programs, agencies, and departments.
- CHI only covers "*existing* health information interoperability standards (health vocabulary and messaging)."
- CHI *already has adopted* 19 of 24 standards.

The implications of these points are, respectively:

- The private healthcare sector is not required to adopt these standards, unlike HIPAA Administrative Simplification. However, as discussed, there are good reasons for doing so.
- The federal government is not going to develop new standards, but will adopt standards that have been developed and are in use and have proven to be beneficial in a variety of healthcare venues.
- The federal government has made considerably more progress with CHI than it has with HIPAA Administrative Simplification, constrained by adoption procedures required under the Administrative Procedures Act. With rising healthcare costs and baby boomers moving into the Medicare program starting in 2011, there is scant time to reinvent clinical vocabularies and messaging protocols that often take considerable time and resources to move through standards adoption processes.

Is the private healthcare sector off the hook with respect to the clinical standards that are being adopted by the federal government? Not likely. The government is leading by example and using its considerable size in the US healthcare sector to *encourage* adoption of the same clinical standards. As noted in the next chapter, the CHI standards will provide the functional content for the electronic health record (EHR) for which the federal government likely will implement provider investment and claim reimbursement incentives for private sector providers to adopt and use. The US is not going to have one system for the public sector and another for the private sector. As Secretary Thompson said, "The private sector will be crucial to the widespread diffusion of these standards."[13]

CONSOLIDATED HEALTH INFORMATICS INITIATIVE

The foundation of the CHI initiative is "the same clinical vocabularies and the same ways of transmitting that information."[14] Vocabulary means *code sets* and transmitting means *messaging*. These are discussed further in the following sidebars, "Focus on Code Sets" and "Focus on Messaging."

Focus on Code Sets[15]

A *code set* is a body of information "used to encode data elements" that is created and maintained by a code set maintaining organization. A code set has predetermined values, which are distinguished from data that would be used to encode data elements based on values drawn, for example, from information about a person such as age.

An example of a code set that is easily recognized is a *zip code*. A zip code directory, created and maintained by the US Postal Service, is a code set from which you would select a predetermined value based on the location of a particular address. For example, if I know an address in Pasadena, California, I can go to the zip code directory, look up the street name, and find the zip code.[16] In contrast, age is a value based on personal knowledge that is self-reported or otherwise imparted to you. Both types of values are critical to implementation of standards and populating underlying data elements.

External code sets are integral to the establishment and use of standards. You are not expected to know vast bodies of information that will facilitate an exchange of information in a transaction. You also are not expected to develop your own description of a place or an event because the other party to a transaction may not understand your description. Think what would happen if instead of using a zip code each person used his or her own location rule or description of an event. For example, the rules that define zip codes are that they have five numeric characters (numbers) and cover the US and zip+4 codes have five numeric characters, a hyphen, and four trailing numeric characters and cover the US. We learn zip code values from a directory or computer file, and everybody uses them.

We learn values that define the numeric characteristic of age at an early age, based on a common understanding of implicit rules. Everybody uses zip codes and everybody defines the numeric characteristic of age in round numbers, say between 1 and 80, but we get the values from different sources.

Focus on Messaging

The "same ways of transmitting" information means that individuals or entities exchanging information "are able to transmit that information in a way that maintains its meaning. This sharing information within and between agencies establishes 'interoperability.'"[14] There are two attributes of interoperability:

■ Ability to have transmitter and receiver communicate using standard communication protocols.

■ Ability to have transmitted information interpreted by receiver exactly as understood by transmitter.

As children, we all played the telephone game in which we sat in a circle, one person thought of a sentence to pass along in a whisper to the next person,

continued

and so on around the circle. All the children laughed when the last person reported what he heard, and the initiator reported what she said, and the two differed markedly.

The healthcare environment today is very similar to that game and its outcome. Frequently, data elements contain or connote different meanings or interpretations. Many providers are unable to communicate electronically because practice management systems use different standards for creating, storing, or transmitting information, or a combination thereof.

It is messaging capabilities, interoperability, that distinguish an EMR from an EHR. The former is physician-centric whereas the latter is patient-centric. An electronic *medical* record may be of value to a physician practice as a tool for more efficiently conducting the business of the practice. That is what we mean by physician-centric. In contrast, an electronic *health* record is of value to a patient because it lets the patient maintain an up-to-date health record by virtue of different providers communicating results to one another following encounters with the patient. Of course, the EHR is of value to the physician as well because it is an efficient tool for delivering services to patients and communicating with other healthcare practitioners. We explore interoperability again in Chapter 6.

On March 21, 2003, HHS, the US Department of Defense, and the US Department of Veterans Affairs "announced the first set of uniform standards for the electronic exchange of clinical health information to be adopted across the federal government."[14] Of the 24 domains comprising the CHI initiative, five were initially adopted. Descriptions for these five domains are drawn from information and links at the CHI Web site at www.whitehouse.gov/omb/egov/downloads/Domain2.doc.

- **Domain: Messaging.**
  - Health Level 7 (HL7) messaging standards to ensure that each federal agency can share information that will improve coordinated care for patients such as entries of orders, scheduling appointments and tests and better coordination of the admittance, discharge, and transfer of patients.[14]
- **Domain: Messaging Standards for Retail Pharmacy Transactions.**
  - National Council for Prescription Drug Programs (NCPDP) standards for ordering drugs from retail pharmacies to standardize information between healthcare providers and the pharmacies. These standards already have been adopted under the Health Insurance Portability and Accountability Act (HIPAA) of 1996, and ensure that parts of the three federal departments that aren't covered by HIPAA will also use the same standards.

    These standards cover electronic transfer of prescription data between retail pharmacies and prescribers for new prescriptions, prescription changes, prescription refill requests, prescription fill status notifications, and cancellation notifications. NCPDP, an approved standards developing organization of the American National Standards Institute (ANSI), owns the standards. Information on acquisition of the standards is available online at www.ncpdp.org.[17]

- **Domain: Messaging Standard for Connectivity.**
  - The Institute of Electrical and Electronics Engineers 1073 (IEEE1073) series of standards that allow for healthcare providers to plug medical devices into information and computer systems that allow healthcare providers to monitor information from an intensive care unit (ICU) or through telehealth services on Indian reservations, and in other circumstances.

    The standard specifically addresses the requirement for two devices to automatically configure a connection for successful operation, independent of connection type. The standard defines a device-to-device internal messaging system within an agency. Work is underway to allow seamless connection to HL7 enabled devices for exchange of information between agencies. The IEEE 1073 General Committee owns the standard and is chartered under the IEEE Engineering in Medicine and Biology Society. Information on acquisition of IEEE standards is available online at www.shop/ieee.org/store.[18]

- **Domain: Messaging Standard for Images That Enable Images and Associated Diagnostic Information to Be Retrieved and Transferred From Various Manufacturers' Devices as Well as Medical Staff Workstations.**
  - Digital Imaging Communications in Medicine (DICOM) standards that enable images and associated diagnostic information to be retrieved and transferred from various manufacturers' devices as well as medical staff workstations. DICOM has two parts:
    - Information objects: how images and image-related information are encoded.
    - Services: how information objects are exchanged between instruments, either on network or on offline media.
  - National Electrical Manufacturers Association (NEMA) owns the copyright to DICOM standards, which are administered by the NEMA Diagnostic Imaging and Therapy Systems Division. Information on acquisition of DICOM standards is available online at www.medical.nema.org.[19]

- **Domain: Laboratory Results Names**
  - Laboratory Logical Observation Identifier Name Codes (LOINC) to standardize the electronic exchange of clinical laboratory results.
  - Lab test ordering and lab test result values are included in standards adopted on May 6, 2004 and discussed later in this chapter. The Regenstrief Institute, Inc. owns LOINC. The LOINC database and

associated documents and programs are copyrighted, but the copyright permits commercial and noncommercial uses in perpetuity at no cost. Information on acquisition of LOINC is available at www.regenstrief.org/LOINC.[20]

On May 6, 2004, HHS, the US Department of Defense, and the US Department of Veterans Affairs adopted 15 additional standards of the 24 domains, making a total of 19 adopted. They are identified here from Secretary Thompson's May 6, 2004, news release and annotated with information from "CHIExec Summaries," a document available for download at the E-Gov Web site at www.whitehouse.gov/omb/egov/downloads/ CHIExecSummaries.doc.[5]

Five of the domains are Health Level 7 (HL7) vocabulary standards for demographic information, units of measure, immunizations, and clinical encounters, and HL7's Clinical Document Architecture standard for test-based reports. HL7 is an ANSI standards developing organization and holds copyrights on the standards described in the five domains below. Information on acquisition of these standards is available online at www.hl7.org.

The five HL7 domains are:

- **Domain: Demographics**
  - HL7 Version 2.4+ standard sets requirements for collecting and storing specific patient demographic data, used primarily for unique patient identification.[21]

- **Domain: Units**
  - HL7 Version 2.X+ standard defines units of measure, such as Celsius or mg/ml, that are intended to be combined with a numeric value to accurately express a result.[22]

- **Domain: Immunizations**
  - HL7 Version 2.3.1+ standard for storage and exchange of immunization data provides an organized and streamlined means of communicating between federal partners by offering a real time means of transferring information regarding immunization encounters, vaccine events, patient records, and other immunization-related information important to immunization registries.[23]

- **Domain: Clinical Encounters**
  - HL7 Version 2.4+ standard serves as a focal point linking clinical, administrative, and financial information for encounters in different settings: ambulatory care, inpatient care, emergency care, home healthcare, field care, and virtual care via telemedicine.[24]

- **Domain: Text Based Reports**
  - HL7 CDA Release 1.0-2000 standards and terminologies define messaging architecture and syntax of clinical text documents.[25]

Five of the domains are College of American Pathologists Systematized Nomenclature of Medicine-Clinical Terms (SNOMED-CT) copyrighted standards for laboratory result contents, non-laboratory interventions and procedures, anatomy, diagnosis and problems, and nursing. HHS is making SNOMED-CT available for use in the United States at no charge to users.[26]

- **Domain: Laboratory Result Contents**
  - This SNOMED-CT standard is used to exchange results of laboratory tests between facilities. The results are contained within a laboratory report that includes additional items such as patient and order demographics, a LOINC code laboratory test name, specimen type, and other items that may be required by business needs or messaging structures.[27]

- **Domain: Non-Laboratory Interventions and Procedures**
  - This SNOMED-CT standard is used to describe specific non-laboratory interventions and procedures performed and delivered. Interventions represent purposeful activities performed in providing healthcare. Procedures conceptually represent purposeful activities performed in providing healthcare.[28]

- **Domain: Anatomy and Physiology**[29]
  - This SNOMED-CT anatomy standard describes anatomical locations for clinical, surgical, pathological, and research purposes.[30]

- **Domain: Diagnosis and Problem Lists**
  - This SNOMED-CT standard broadly defines a series of brief statements that catalog a patient's medical, nursing, dental, social, preventive, and psychiatric events and issues that are relevant to that patient's healthcare, such as signs, symptoms, and defined conditions.[31]

- **Domain: Nursing**
  - This SNOMED-CT standard defines terminology that is used to identify, classify, and name the delivery of nursing care. Sub-domains are derived from the Nursing Process and American Nursing Association (ANA) recognized Nursing Minimum Data Set (NMDS), which emphasizes nursing assessment, diagnosis, interventions, and outcomes of nursing care.[32]

The next two domains represent individual CHI standards.

- **Domain: Interventions and Procedures, Laboratory Test Order Names**
  - Laboratory Logical Observation Identifier Name Codes (LOINC) standardize electronic exchange of laboratory test orders and drug label section headers, and represent here names of laboratory tests associated with an order in a computer system. Excluded from this standard, but embodied in other CHI standards, are laboratory results naming, laboratory test result values, demographics, anatomy, genes, and proteins. The Regenstrief Institute, Inc. owns LOINC. The LOINC database and associated documents and programs are copyrighted, but the copyright permits commercial and noncommercial uses in perpetuity at no cost. Information on acquisition of LOINC is available at www. regenstrief.org/LOINC.[33]

- **Domain: Billing/Financial**

  - Health Insurance Portability and Accountability Act (HIPAA)[34] Administration Simplification transactions and code sets cover electronic exchange of health related information to perform billing or administrative functions. These are the same standards now required under HIPAA for health plans, healthcare clearinghouses and those healthcare providers who engage in certain electronic transactions. For the CHI Billing/Financial domain, the transaction and code set standards that are part of HIPAA Administrative Simplification represent one billing/financial standard.

  - Transaction and Code Set Standards. The transaction standards required compliance by health plans, healthcare clearinghouses, and healthcare providers that initiated electronic transactions on or after October 16, 2003.[35] The descriptions of the transactions that follow focus on titles of NCPDP and Accredited Standards Committee (ASC) X12N implementation guides and addenda associated with each transaction standard. Implementation guides and addenda for X12N standards are available from Washington Publishing Company (WPC) at www.wpc-edi.com.[36] Code sets are beyond the scope of discussion here, but are described for each transaction standard in the respective implementation guides.[37] Information on National Council for Prescription Drug Programs (NCPDP) implementation guides is available in portable document format (pdf) at www.ncpdp.org/PDF/batchstandard.pdf.[38]

HIPAA Administrative Simplification Transaction Standards

Health claims or equivalent encounter information

- Retail pharmacy drug claims
  - National Council for Prescription Drug Programs (NCPDP) Telecommunication Standard Implementation Guide, Version 5, Release 1 (Version 5.1), September 1999, and equivalent NCPDP Batch Implementation Guide, Version 1, Release 1 (Version 1.1), January 2000, in support of Telecommunication Standard Implementation Guide, Version 5.1, for the NCPDP Data Record in the Detail Data Record.
- Dental healthcare claim
  - Accredited Standards Committee (ASC) X12N 837—Healthcare Claim: Dental, Version 4010, May 2000, Washington Publishing Company (WPC), 004010X097, and Addenda to Healthcare Claim: Dental, Version 4010, October 2002, WPC, 004010X097A1.[39]
- Professional healthcare claim
  - ASC X12N 837—Healthcare Claim: Professional, Volumes 1 and 2, Version 4010, May 2000, WPC, 004010X098, and Addenda to Healthcare

Claim: Professional, Volumes 1 and 2, Version 4010, October 2002, WPC, 004010X098A1.

- Institutional healthcare claim
  - ASC X12N 837—Healthcare Claim: Institutional, Volumes 1 and 2, Version 4010, May 2000, WPC, 004010X096, and Addenda to Healthcare Claim: Institutional, Volumes 1 and 2, Version 4010, October 2002, WPC, 004010X096A1.

Enrollment and disenrollment in a health plan

- ASC X12N 834: Benefit Enrollment and Maintenance, Version 4010, May 2000, WPC, 004010X095, and Addenda to Benefit Enrollment and Maintenance, Version 4010, October 2002, WPC, 004010X095A1.

Eligibility for a health plan

- Dental, professional, institutional healthcare eligibility benefit inquiry and response
  - ASC X12N 270/271: Healthcare Eligibility Benefit Inquiry and Response, Version 4010, May 2000, WPC, 004010X092, and Addenda to Healthcare Eligibility Benefit Inquiry and Response, Version 4010, October 2002, WPC, 004010X092A1.
- Retail pharmacy drugs
  - NCPDP Telecommunication Standard Implementation Guide, Version 5.1, September 1999, and equivalent NCPDP Batch Implementation Guide, Version 1.1, January 2000, in support of Telecommunication Standard Implementation Guide, Version 5.1, for the NCPDP Data Record in the Detail Data Record.

Healthcare payment and remittance advice

- ASC X12N 835: Healthcare Claim Payment/Advice, Version 4010, May 2000, WPC, 004010X091, and Addenda to Healthcare Claim Payment/Advice, Version 4010, October 2002, WPC, 004010X091A1.

Health plan premium payments

- ASC X12N 820: Payroll Deducted and Other Group Premium Payment for Insurance Products, Version 4010, May 2000, WPC, 004010X061, and Addenda to Payroll Deducted and Other Group Premium Payment for Insurance Products, Version 4010, October 2002, WPC, 004010X061A1.

Health claim status

- ASC X12N 276/277: Healthcare Claim Status Request and Response, Version 4010, May 2000, WPC, 004010X093A1, and Addenda to Healthcare

continued

Claim Status Request and Response, Version 4010, October 2002, 004010X093A1.

Referral certification and authorization

- Dental, professional, institutional referral certification and authorization

    - ASC X12N 278: Healthcare Services Review—Request for Review and Response, Version 4010, May 2000, WPC, 004010X094, and Addenda to Healthcare Services Review—Request for Review and Response, Version 4010, October 2002, WPC, 004010X094A1.

- Retail pharmacy drug referral certification and authorization

    - NCPDP Telecommunication Standard Implementation Guide, Version 5.1, September 1999, and equivalent NCPDP Batch Implementation Guide, Version 1.1, January 2000, in support of Telecommunication Standard Implementation Guide, Version 5.1, for the NCPDP Data Record in the Detail Data Record.

Coordination of benefits information[40]

- Retail pharmacy drug claim

    - NCPDP Telecommunication Standard Implementation Guide, Version 5.1, September 1999, and equivalent NCPDP Batch Implementation Guide, Version 1.1, January 2000, in support of Telecommunication Standard Implementation Guide, Version 5.1, for the NCPDP Data Record in the Detail Data Record.

- Dental healthcare claim

    - Accredited Standards Committee (ASC) X12N 837—Healthcare Claim: Dental, Version 4010, May 2000, Washington Publishing Company (WPC), 004010X097, and Addenda to Healthcare Claim: Dental, Version 4010, October 2002, WPC, 004010X097A1.

- Professional healthcare claim

    - ASC X12N 837—Healthcare Claim: Professional, Volumes 1 and 2, Version 4010, May 2000, WPC, 004010X098, and Addenda to Healthcare Claim: Professional, Volumes 1 and 2, Version 4010, October 2002, WPC, 004010X098A1.

- Institutional healthcare claim

    - ASC X12N 837—Healthcare Claim: Institutional, Volumes 1 and 2, Version 4010, May 2000, WPC, 004010X096, and Addenda to Healthcare Claim: Institutional, Volumes 1 and 2, Version 4010, October 2002, WPC, 004010X096A1.

The next domain, Medications, comprises six subdomains that represent one CHI standard.

These subdomains are a set of federal terminologies related to medications, including the Food and Drug Administration's names and codes for ingredients, manufactured dosage forms, drug products and medication packages, the National Library of Medicine's RxNORM for describing clinical drugs, and the Veterans Administration's National Drug File Reference Terminology (NDF-RT) for specific drug classifications.

■ **Domain: Medications; Sub-Domain: Active Ingredients**
   ■ The Food and Drug Administration (FDA) Established Name for Active Ingredient and Unique Ingredient Identifier (UNII) codes standard enables the federal healthcare sector to share information regarding medication active ingredients. An active ingredient is a substance responsible for the effects of a medication. Frequently, an active ingredient is a known chemical substance. In certain instances, the structure of an ingredient may not be known precisely. These FDA standard names and codes are in the public domain, and administered by FDA. Information on them is available at www.fda.gov.[41]

■ **Domain: Medications; Sub-Domain: Manufactured Dosage Form**
   ■ The FDA/Center for Drug Evaluation and Research (CDER) Data Standards Manual enables the federal health sector to share information regarding drug dosage forms. A manufactured dosage form is the way of identifying the drug in its physical form. In determining dosage form, FDA examines such factors as:
      ■ Physical appearance of the drug product.
      ■ Physical form of the drug product prior to dispensing to the patient.
      ■ The way the drug is administered.
      ■ Frequency of dosing.
      ■ How pharmacists and other health professionals might recognize and handle drug products.
   ■ Dosage form terms are in the public domain, and available online at FDA's CDER Web site at: www.fda.gov/cder/dsm/DRG/drg00201.htm.[42]

■ **Domain: Medications; Sub-Domain: Drug Product**
   ■ FDA's National Drug Code (NDC) enables the federal healthcare sector to share information regarding drug products. The NDC list of products and their codes is available without a licensing agreement, and can be accessed online at: www.fda.gov/cder/ndc/index.htm.[43]

■ **Domain: Medications; Sub-Domain: Package**
   ■ The FDA/CDER Data Standards Manual enables the federal health sector to share information regarding drug packages. Package terms are in the public domain, and are available online at: www.fda.gov/cder/dsm/drg/drg00907.htm.[44]

■ **Domain: Medications; Sub-Domain: Clinical Drug[45]**
   ■ The Semantic Clinical Drug (SCD) of RxNorm standard enables the federal healthcare sector to share information regarding medication

active ingredients. The National Library of Medicine has primary responsibility for RxNorm terminology, which is a public domain system developed by the National Library of Medicine with the Veterans Administration and FDA, in consultation with HL7. RxNorm is distributed by the Unified Medical Language System (UMLS) without restriction, and information on RxNorm is available online at: www.nim.nih.gov/research/umls.[46]

■ **Domain: Medications; Sub-Domain: Drug Classifications**

■ The National Drug File Reference Terminology (NDF-RT) is a classification scheme for the areas of Physiologic Effect and Mechanism of Action. This standardized medication terminology includes hierarchical structures for categorizing each medication, such as mechanism of action, physiologic effects, intended therapeutic use, chemical structures, pharmacological properties, and FDA approved indications. The Veterans Administration developed NDF-RT, which may be obtained from the VA or online from the National Cancer Institute at: www.nciterms.nci.hih.gov/ncibrowser/connect.do.[47]

The last two CHI standards that were approved in May 2004 follow.

■ **Domain: Genes and Proteins**

■ The Human Gene Nomenclature (HUGN) is for exchanging information regarding the role of genes in biomedical research in the federal health sector.[48] Protein nomenclature is not included in the standard. HUGN is sponsored by the Human Genome Organization (HUGO), a nonprofit entity jointly funded by the United Kingdom Medical Research Council and the US National Institutes of Health. HUGN is free for nonprofit use, but requires a license for commercial use. Information on HUGN is available at: www.gene.ucl.ac.uk/nomenclature/information/commercial.html.

■ **Domain: Chemicals**

■ The Environmental Protection Agency's (EPA) Substance Registry System[49] covers non-medicinal chemicals of importance to healthcare.[50] These chemicals likely will be found in the workplace or in the environment that are related to health issues. For example, a use of the chemical code might be during a "first encounter and perhaps be part of a History and Physical." EPA's Substance Registry System is free and does not require a license for use. Information on the Substance Registry System is available on EPA's Environmental Metadata Gateway (EMG) at: www.epa.gov/emg.

The CHI program is considering adopting five more standards in the future in the following domains:

■ History and physical
■ Disability
■ Medical devices and supplies

- Population health
- Multimedia

Progress on adoption of these standards can be monitored on the E-Gov Web site at: www.whitehouse.gov/omb/egov/gtob/health_informatics.htm.

SUMMARY

In this chapter we outlined the federal Consolidated Health Informatics initiative, which applies to federal agencies that are involved in healthcare activities. The CHI initiative is a change from the HIPAA Administrative Simplification standards that were implemented pursuant to the Administrative Procedures Act. The HIPAA Administrative Simplification standards have taken longer to implement than the enabling legislation anticipated. As a result, the CHI initiatives, which encompass clinical as well as administrative standards, are designed to implement standards more quickly and to serve as examples for the private healthcare sector to adopt, most likely with federal incentives.

In Chapter 6, we examine the recently adopted HL7 EHR draft standards for trial use. You will see how many of these CHI standards are integral to its successful implementation and use.

ENDNOTES

1. Quoted in: Murphy-Barron C, Parke R, Sander M. Is there an actuary in the house? *Contingencies*. July/August 2004, p 45.
2. These administrative standards are discussed in two of our books that were published by AMA Press in 2004: *HIPAA Plain & Simple: A Compliance Guide for Healthcare Professionals* and *HIPAA Transactions: A Nontechnical Business Guide for Healthcare.*
3. See *Presidential Statement*, available on the White House Web site at: www.whitehouse.gov/omb/egov/pres_state.htm
4. US Department of Health and Human Services. "HHS Launches New Efforts to Promote Paperless Healthcare System," news release, Tuesday, July 1, 2003. Available at: www.hhs.gov/news/press/2003pres/20030701.html.
5. US Department of Health and Human Services. "Secretary Thompson, Seeking Fastest Possible Results, Names First Health Information Technology Coordinator," news release, Thursday, May 6, 2004. Available at: www.hhs.gov/news/press/2004pres/20040506.html.
6. US Department of Health and Human Services. "The Decade of Health Information Technology: Delivering Consumer-Centric and Information-Rich Healthcare," fact sheet, Wednesday, July 21, 2004. Available at: www.hhs.gov/news.
7. Health Level Seven, Inc. "HL7 Board of Directors Unanimously Approves EHR for Draft Standard Status; New EHR Ballot Numbers Released as Reconciliation Continues," press release, July 27, 2004. Available at: www.hl7.org.

8. *About E-Gov*, available on the White House Web site at: www.whitehouse. gov/omb/egov/about_backgrnd.htm.

9. An online description of this law is available at: www.whitehouse.gov/omb/egov/pres_state2.htm.

10 Goedert J. What's in a name? Perhaps the future of IT. *Health Data Management.* December 22, 2004. Available at: www.healthdatamanagement.com/HDMSearchResultsDetails.cfm?DID=13554.

11. For attributes of all E-Gov initiatives and updates, when available, go to the White House Web site at: www.whitehouse.gov/omb/egov/downloads/ e-gov_initiatives.htm.

12. An example is the federal government's licensing of the Systematized Nomenclature of Medicine-Clinical Terms (SNOMED-CT), which is owned by the College of American Pathologists.

13. "Federal Government Announces First Federal E-Gov Health Information Exchange Standards," press release, March 21, 2003. Available at: www.whitehouse.gov/omb/egov/press/chi_march.htm.

14. For more information, see www.whitehouse.gov/omb/egov/downloads/ Domain2.doc.

15. Reprinted from Jones ED III, Hartley CP. *HIPAA Transactions: A Nontechnical Business Guide for Healthcare.* Chicago, Ill: AMA Press; 2004:59–60.

16. For example, at the Web site, www.usps.gov, I can click on "Find a Zip Code," enter the house number, street address, city, and state, and get a Zip+4 code in response.

17. See www.whitehouse.gov/omb/egov/downloads/Doman3.doc

18. See www.whitehouse.gov/omb/egov/downloads/Doman4.doc

19. See www.whitehouse.gov/omb/egov/downloads/Doman5.doc

20. See www.whitehouse.gov/omb/egov/downloads/Doman1.doc

21. CHIExecSummaries, p 14.

22. CHIExecSummaries, p 13.

23. CHIExecSummaries, p 11. This standard is available for any healthcare organization to use without a use license. An implementation guide for immunization data transactions is available online at the National Immunization Program Web site at: www.cdc.gov/nip/registry.

24. CHIExecSummaries, p 7.

25. CHIExecSummaries, p 27.

26. Secretary Thompson made the following announcement on May 6, 2004, with regard to SNOMED-CT: SNOMED-CT "is now available for download as part of the National Library of Medicine's Unified Medical Language System (UMLS) Metathesaurus at www.umlsinfor.nim.hih.gov. The vocabulary is available free for anyone in the US. Users must register via the Web for a free UMLS license before downloading the data or requesting a copy on DVD. With terms for more than 300,000 current medical concepts, the College's standardized system has been recognized as the world's most comprehensive clinical terminology database available. . . . It is now possible for healthcare providers, hospitals, insurance companies, public health departments, medical research facilities, and others to easily incorporate this uniform terminology

system into their information systems." US Department of Health and Human Services. "Secretary Thompson, Seeking Fastest Possible Results, Names First Health Information Technology Coordinator," news release, Thursday, May 6, 2004. Available at: www.hhs.gov/news/press/2004pres/20040506.html.

27. CHIExecSummaries, p 12.

28. CHIExecSummaries, p 10.

29. There is no standard for physiology recommended under the Consolidated Health Informatics program.

30. CHIExecSummaries, p 1.

31. CHIExecSummaries, p 6.

32. CHIExecSummaries, p 24.

33. CHIExecSummaries, p 14.

34. Public Law 104-191, enacted in August 1996. Information on HIPAA and final regulatory rules available at: www.cms.hhs.gov/hipaa/hipaa2.

35. Department of Health and Human Services, Office of the Secretary. "45 CFR Part 162: Health Insurance Reform: Modifications to Electronic Data Transaction Standards and Code Sets; Final Rule." *Federal Register.* v 68, n 34, February 20, 2003, pp 8381–8399; and "Correction." *Federal Register.* v 68, n 46, p 11445.

36. Go to Washington Publishing Company's Web site, as noted in the text, click on "HIPAA," and then on "Implementation Guides." You will have to register with WPC in order to download the implementation guides and addenda in portable document format (pdf) at no charge. The total numbers of implementation guide and addenda pages are 3696 and 526 pages, respectively, which will eat up over eight reams of paper and lots of computer download time. As an alternative, you may prefer to purchase a paper bound copy or pdf version on diskette of the implementation guides and addenda, which you can do online or by calling WPC at 800-972-4334.

37. External code sets for the transaction guides are summarized in Table 4.1 in Jones ED III, Hartley CP. *HIPAA Transactions: A Nontechnical Business Guide for Healthcare.* Chicago, Ill: AMA Press; 2004:65–67.

38. To download a free copy of Adobe® Reader® software for viewing and printing portable document format (PDF) documents, go to www.adobe.com/products/acraobat/readstep2.html.

39. The version is "4010" for each of the standards. This version is based on work done by members of Accredited Standards Committee (ASC) X12 on standards. Whether "4010" or "004010," the notation refers to version 4, release 1, subrelease 0. Although newer versions are being used in other industries, version 4010 provides a baseline for healthcare stakeholders to implement EDI standards using a common set of data formats and data content. Each standard has two notations, one of which is an "addendum." The addenda provide some modification of original data content based on a better understanding of the use of specified information in business transactions. A comprehensive discussion of the X12 Administrative Simplification transaction standards is in *HIPAA Transactions: A Nontechnical Business Guide for Healthcare* by Edward D. Jones III and Carolyn P. Hartley (AMA Press, 2004).

40. The two transactions standards, *Health claims or equivalent encounter information* and *Coordination of benefits information,* use the same NCPDP and ASC X12N implementation guides.
41. CHIExec Summaries, p 19.
42. CHIExec Summaries, p 18.
43. CHIExec Summaries, p 21.
44. CHIExec Summaries, p 20.
45. CHIExecSummaries, p 15. "A 'clinical drug' is a name for a pharmaceutical preparation consisting of its component(s), defined as active ingredients and their strength, together with the dose form of the drug as given to the patient. It expresses the equivalence of pharmaceutical preparations at a generic level, in the form in which medications are prescribed for the patient."
46. CHIExec Summaries, p 15.
47. CHIExec Summaries, p 17.
48. CHIExecSummaries, p 8.
49. This is EPA's central system for information concerning regulated and monitored substances.
50. ChiExecSummaries, p 3.

chapter 6

Electronic Health Record Systems: The Health Level Seven Draft Standards for Trial Use

In this chapter, we describe the Health Level Seven (HL7) electronic health record draft standard for trial use (EHR-DSTU). You will recall from Chapter 5 that in July 2003, the federal government provided the impetus for moving the industry more quickly to standards pertaining to electronic health records (EHRs), including more rapid adoption of clinical vocabularies that would facilitate interoperability, or communication of medical information among practitioners and between practitioners and patients.

The initiation of the two-year test phase of the EHR-DTSU coincided with Secretary of Health and Human Services (HHS) Tommy Thompson's launch of the "Decade of Health Information Technology" in July 2004[1] at the *Secretarial Summit on Health Information Technology* in Washington, DC.[2]

WHAT YOU WILL LEARN IN THIS CHAPTER

- Four goals and 12 strategies of Secretary Thompson's "Decade of Health Information Technology"
- The functional descriptors that compose HL7's EHR-DSTU
- How to communicate your comments on the EHR-DSTU functional descriptors to HL7

Key Terms

EHR-DSTU: The electronic health record draft standard for trial use, which is defined and managed by Health Level Seven.
Functional Descriptor: A component of the EHR-DSTU that identifies, describes, rationalizes, and provides a foundation for its use.

THE DECADE OF HEALTH INFORMATION TECHNOLOGY

Secretary Thompson's July 21, 2004 launch of the "Decade of Health Information Technology" reflects the federal government's policy shift from administrative to clinical standards that we discussed in Chapter 5. Several months earlier, on May 6, 2004, Secretary Thompson announced the appointment of David Brailer, MD, PhD, as the National Health Information Coordinator to coordinate and facilitate the implementation of the policy.[3] Secretary Thompson stated that the focus of the policy was to "transform the delivery of healthcare by building a new health information infrastructure, including electronic health records and a new network to link health records nationwide."[1] To support this effort, the Secretary listed four goals and 12 strategies, primarily on the clinical side. These are reproduced here[2]:

- **Goal 1: *Inform Clinical Practice*.** This goal centers largely around effort to bring EHRs directly into clinical practice.
  - **Strategy 1: *Provide Incentives for EHR Adoption*.** The transition to safe, more consumer-friendly and regionally integrated care delivery will require shared investments in information tools and changes to current clinical practice.
  - **Strategy 2: *Reduce Risk of EHR Investment*.** Clinicians who purchase EHRs and who attempt to change their clinical practices and office operations face a variety of risks that make this decision unduly challenging. Low-cost support systems that reduce risk, failure, and partial use of EHRs are needed.
  - **Strategy 3: *Promote EHR Diffusion in Rural and Underserved Areas*.** Practices and hospitals in rural and other underserved areas lag in EHR adoption. Technology transfer and other support efforts are needed to ensure widespread adoption.
- **Goal 2: *Interconnect Clinicians*.** Interconnecting clinicians will allow information to be portable and to move with consumers from one point of care to another. This will require an interoperable infrastructure to help clinicians get access to critical healthcare information when their clinical and/or treatment decisions are being made.
  - **Strategy 1: *Regional Collaborations*.** Local oversight of health information exchange that reflects the needs and goals of a population should be developed.
  - **Strategy 2: *Develop a National Health Information Network*.** A set of common intercommunication tools such as mobile authentication, Web services architecture, and security technologies is needed to support data movement that is inexpensive and secure. A national health information network that can provide low-cost and secure data

movement is needed, along with public-private oversight or management function to ensure adherence to public policy objectives.

- **Strategy 3:** *Coordinate Federal Health Information Systems.* There is a need for federal health information systems to be interoperable and to exchange data so that federal care delivery, reimbursement, and oversight are more efficient and cost-effective. Federal health information systems will be interoperable and consistent with the national health information network.

- **Goal 3:** *Personalize Care.* Consumer-centric information helps individuals manage their own wellness and assists with their personal healthcare decisions.

  - **Strategy 1:** *Encourage Use of Personal Health Records (PHRs).* Consumers are increasing seeking information about their care as a means of getting better control over their healthcare experience, and PHRs that provide customized facts and guidance to them are needed.

  - **Strategy 2:** *Enhance Informed Consumer Choice.* Consumers should have the ability to select clinicians and institutions based on what they value and the information to guide their choice, including the quality of care providers deliver.

  - **Strategy 3:** *Promote Use of Telehealth Systems.* The use of telehealth—remote communication technologies—can provide access to health services for consumers and clinicians in rural and underserved areas.

- **Goal 4:** *Improve Population Health.* Population health improvement envisions improved capacity for public health monitoring, quality of care measurement, and bringing research advance more quickly into medical practice.

  - **Strategy 1:** *Unify Public Health Surveillance Architectures.* An interoperable public health surveillance system is needed that will allow exchange of information, consistent with privacy laws, to better protect against disease.

  - **Strategy 2:** *Streamline Quality and Health Status Monitoring.* Many different state and local organizations collect subsets of data for specific purposes and use it in different ways. A streamlined quality-monitoring infrastructure that will allow a complete look at quality and other issues in real-time and at the point of care is needed.

  - **Strategy 3:** *Accelerate Research and Dissemination of Evidence.* Information tools are needed that can accelerate scientific discoveries and their translation into clinically useful products, applications, and knowledge.

It is important for physicians to note that federal clinical initiatives are *voluntary*, unlike their administrative counterparts, the Health Insurance

Portability and Accountability Act of 1996 (HIPAA) Administrative Simplification standards, which are *mandatory*. As the goals and strategies suggest, the federal government is going to provide incentives for healthcare providers to use interoperable, certified EHRs that embody and integrate electronic administrative functionality. We shall see that in the *supportive* functional descriptors of the EHR-DSTU, which follows. The voluntary clinical initiatives could not be supported without the mandatory privacy and security protections offered by the HIPAA Administrative Simplification standards.

HEALTH LEVEL SEVEN'S DRAFT STANDARD ELECTRONIC HEALTH RECORD

Today, most medical records are constructed on paper and maintained in paper file systems in physician practices, hospitals, dental practices, other healthcare service facilities, health plans, and patient files. Parts of these records may be kept as electronic data files on computer systems. However, when a caregiver, health plan, or patient seeks information from a medical record, it generally is in a paper format and scattered among the patient's caregivers, health plans, and the patient's own files.

In the healthcare industry, with a projected national expenditure of more than $1.79 trillion in 2004,[4] that is a lot of paper and a lot of files. In an era of mobility for work and leisure, it is difficult for caregivers to access useful medical information from records that are scattered about, likely incomplete, and updated only occasionally, if at all.

In the wake of September 11, 2001, the anthrax threat later that year, and the severe acute respiratory syndrome (SARS) epidemic in late 2002, the federal government focused attention on the way in which medical records have been created and maintained. It determined that the current paper-based system was inadequate for government and healthcare industry response to public health threats. Further, the way in which the healthcare industry dealt with medical records was insufficient for identifying and mitigating medical errors, detecting potentially injurious or fatal drug interactions, and accessing critical medical record information in a personal medical emergency.

To remedy these deficiencies, Secretary of HHS Tommy Thompson announced on July 1, 2003, that HHS had commissioned the Institute of Medicine to design a model of an EHR system and requested HL7[5] to produce a DSTU. After approval of the balloted EHR initiative by HL7 in March 2004, HL7 initiated a two-year pilot testing phase of the EHR-DSTU under auspices of the American National Standards Institute (ANSI) on July 27, 2004. It is important to recognize that the EHR-DSTU is not:

■ A messaging specification

■ An implementation specification

- A conformance specification
- An EHR specification
- A conformance testing metric
- An exercise in creating a definition for an EHR or EHR system[6]

PHYSICIAN INPUT INTO THE ELECTRONIC HEALTH RECORD MODEL

The standards included in this chapter have been translated from technical graphs into narrative form with permission for use granted by HL7. This will give you an idea of what each standard will mean and how you would use it if it becomes the final standard.

It's not often that physicians are invited to *vote* on specific standards. But that's exactly what HL7 hopes you'll do after reading and studying this chapter. For example, you may agree with standards described in the Direct Care section, but your practice has set a new gold standard of how it measures and analyzes reports or tracks clinical research. HL7 would like to know that, and how what your practice has experienced further improves the definition of the EHR functional descriptors. The best time for you to influence the outcome of those standards, not only on your practice, but also on other physician practices with which you share patient or practice information, is while the standards are in draft stage (2004–2006).

Directions for Physician Input

In front of each standard is a small box that you can mark if this standard applies to your practice. Later, you may wish to review these standards and provide comments on them to HL7. The HL7 recommends you use the following link to make comments.

To access the draft standards for trial use (DSTU) document online, go to: www.hl7.org/ehr/downloads/index.asp.

To access the database for collecting comments on the DSTU, go to: www.hl7.org/dstucomments/showdetail.cfm?dstuid=5.

FUNCTIONAL AREAS OF THE ELECTRONIC HEALTH RECORD SYSTEM

Direct Care

- Care Management (DC 1.0)
- Clinical Decision Support (DC 2.0)
- Operations Management and Communication (DC 3.0)

Supportive

- Clinical Support (S 1.0)
- Measurement, Analysis, Research, and Reports (S 2.0)
- Administrative and Financial (S 3.0)

Information Infrastructure

- EHR Security (I 1.0)
- EHR Information and Records Management (I 2.0)
- Unique Identity, Registry, and Directory Services (I 3.0)
- Health Informatics and Terminology Standards (I 4.0)
- Standards-Based Interoperability (I 5.0)
- Business Rules Management (I 6.0)
- Workflow Management (I 7.0)

DIRECT CARE

Care Management (DC 1.0)

Health Information Capture, Management, and Review (DC 1.1)[7]

For those functions related to data capture, data may be captured using standardized code sets or nomenclature, depending on the nature of the data, or captured as unstructured data. Data dependent on care setting are entered by a variety of caregivers. Details of who entered data and when it was captured should be tracked. Data may also be captured from devices or other telehealth applications.

☐ **Identify and Maintain a Patient Record (DC 1.1.1)**
Identify and maintain a single patient record for each patient. Key identifying information is stored and linked to the patient record. Static data elements as well as data elements that will change over time are maintained. A lookup function uses this information to uniquely identify the patient.

☐ **Manage Patient Demographics (DC 1.1.2)**
Capture and maintain demographic information. Where appropriate, the data should be clinically relevant, reportable, and traceable over time. Contact information including addresses and phone numbers, as well as key demographic information such as date of birth, sex, and other information is stored and maintained for reporting purposes and for the provision of care.

☐ **Manage Summary Lists (DC 1.1.3)**
Create and maintain patient-specific summary lists that are structured and coded where appropriate. Patient summary lists can be created from patient-specific data and displayed and maintained in a summary

format. The three functions that follow are important but do not exhaust the possibilities.

☐ **Manage Problem List (DC 1.1.3.1)**
Create and maintain patient-specific problem lists. A problem list may include, but is not limited to: chronic conditions, diagnoses, or symptoms; functional limitations; visit or stay-specific conditions, diagnoses, or symptoms. Problem lists are managed over time, whether over the course of a visit, stay, or lifetime of a patient, allowing documentation of historical information and tracking the changing character of problem(s) and its priority. All pertinent dates, including date noted or diagnosed, dates of any changes in problem specification or prioritization, and date of resolution, are stored. This might include time stamps, where useful and appropriate. The entire problem history for any problem in the list is viewable.

☐ **Manage Medication List (DC 1.1.3.2)**
Create and maintain patient-specific medication lists. Medication lists are managed over time, whether over the course of a visit, stay, or lifetime of a patient. All pertinent dates, including medication start, modification, and end dates, are stored. The entire medication history for any medication, including alternative supplements and herbal medications, is viewable. Medications lists are not limited to medication orders recorded by providers but may include, for example, pharmacy dispense/supply records and patient-recorded medications.

☐ **Manage Allergy and Adverse Reaction List (DC 1.1.3.3)**
Create and maintain patient-specific allergy and adverse reaction lists. Allergens, including immunizations, and substances are identified and coded (whenever possible), and the list is managed over time. All pertinent dates, including patient-reported events, are stored and the description of the patient allergy and adverse reaction is modifiable over time. The entire allergy history, including reaction, for any allergen is viewable. The list(s) includes drug reactions that are not classifiable as a true allergy and intolerances to dietary or environmental triggers. Notations indicating whether item is patient reported and/or provider verified are supported.

☐ ***Manage Patient History (DC 1.1.4)**
Capture, review, and manage medical procedural/surgical, social, and family history, including the capture of pertinent positive and negative histories, and patient-reported or externally available patient clinical history.* The history of the current illness and patient historical data related to previous medical diagnoses, surgeries, and other procedures performed on the patient and relevant health conditions of family members are captured through such methods as patient reporting (eg, interview

or medical alert band) or electronic or nonelectronic historical data. This information may take the form of a positive or a negative, such as: "The patient/family member has had. . . ," or "The patient/family member has not had. . . ." When seen by a healthcare provider, patients typically bring with them clinical information from past encounters. This and similar data are captured and presented alongside locally captured documentation and notes wherever appropriate.

☐ ***Summarize Health Record (DC 1.1.5)***
Present a chronological, filterable, and comprehensive review of a patient's EHR, which may be summarized, subject to privacy and confidentiality requirements. A key feature of an electronic health record is its ability to present, summarize, filter, and facilitate searching through the large amounts of data collected during the provision of patient care. Much of this data is date or date-range specific and should be presented chronologically. Local confidentiality rules that prohibit certain users from accessing certain patient information must be supported.[8]

☐ ***Manage Clinical Documents and Notes (DC 1.1.6)***
Create, addend, correct, authenticate, and close, as needed, transcribed or directly entered clinical documentation and notes. Clinical documents and notes may be created in a narrative form, which may be based on a template. The documents may also be structured documents that result in the capture of coded data. Each form of clinical documentation is important and appropriate for different users and situations.

☐ ***Capture External Clinical Documents (DC 1.1.7)***
Incorporate clinical documentation from external sources. Mechanisms for incorporating external clinical documentation (including identification of source) such as image documents and other clinically relevant data are available. Data incorporated through these mechanisms are presented alongside locally captured documentation and notes wherever appropriate.

☐ ***Capture Patient-Originated Data (DC 1.1.8)***
Capture and explicitly label patient-provided and patient-entered clinical data and support provider authentication for inclusion in patient history. It is critically important to be able to distinguish patient-provided and patient-entered data from clinically authenticated data. Patients may provide data for entry into the health record or be given a mechanism for entering these data directly. Patient-entered data intended for use by care providers will be available for their use.

☐ ***Capture Patient and Family Preferences (DC 1.1.9)***
Capture patient and family preferences at the point of care. Patient and family preferences regarding issues such as language, religion, culture, etc, may be important to the delivery of care. It is important to capture these at the point of care so that they will be available to the provider.

Care Plans, Guidelines, and Protocols (DC 1.2)

☐ ***Present Care Plans, Guidelines, and Protocols (DC 1.2.1)***
Present organization guidelines for patient care as appropriate to support order entry and clinical documentation. Care plans, guidelines, and protocols may be site specific, community or industry-wide standards. They may need to be managed across one or more providers. Tracking of implementation or approval dates, modifications, and relevancy to specific domains or context is provided.

☐ ***Manage Guidelines, Protocols, and Patient-Specific Care Plans (DC 1.2.2)***
Provide administrative tools for organizations to build care plans, guidelines, and protocols for use during patient care planning and care. Guidelines or protocols may contain goals or targets for the patient, specific guidance to the providers, suggested orders, and nursing interventions, among other items.

☐ ***Generate and Record Patient-Specific Instructions (DC 1.2.3)***
Generate and record patient-specific instructions related to pre- and post-procedural and post-discharge requirements. When a patient is scheduled for a test, procedure, or discharge, specific instructions about diet, clothing, transportation assistance, convalescence, follow-up with physician, etc, may be generated and recorded, including the timing relative to the scheduled event.

Medication Ordering and Management (DC 1.3)

☐ ***Order Medication (DC 1.3.1)***
Create prescriptions or other medication orders with detail adequate for correct filling and administration. Provide information regarding compliance of medication orders with formularies. Different medication orders, including discontinue, refill, and renew, require different levels and kinds of detail, as do medication orders placed in different situations. The correct details are recorded for each situation. Administration or patient instructions are available for selection by the ordering clinicians or the ordering clinician is facilitated in creating such instructions. Appropriate time stamps for all medication-related activity are generated. This includes series of orders that are part of a therapeutic regimen, eg, renal dialysis and oncology. When a clinician places an order for a medication, that order may or may not comply with a formulary specific to the patient's location or insurance coverage, if applicable. Whether the order complies with the formulary should be communicated to the ordering clinician at an appropriate point to allow the ordering clinician to decide whether to continue with the order. Formulary-compliant alternatives to the medication being ordered may also be presented.

☐ *Manage Medication Administration (DC 1.3.2)*
Present to appropriate clinicians the list of medications that are to be administered to a patient, under what circumstances, and capture administration details. . . Specifies which medication orders are to be administered by a clinician rather than the patient, the necessary information is presented, including: the list of medication orders that are to be administered; administration instructions, times, or other conditions of administration; dose and route; etc. Additionally, the clinician is able to record what actually was or was not administered, whether or not these facts conform to the order. Appropriate time stamps for all medication-related activity are generated.

Orders, Referrals, and Results Management (DC 1.4)

☐ *Place Patient Care Orders (DC 1.4.1)*
Capture and track orders based on input from specific care providers. Orders that request actions or items can be captured and tracked. Examples include orders to transfer a patient between units; to ambulate a patient; and for medical supplies, durable medical equipment, home IV, and diet or therapy orders. For each orderable item, the appropriate detail, including order identification and instructions, can be captured. Orders should be communicated to the correct recipient for completion if appropriate.

☐ *Order Diagnostic Tests (DC 1.4.2)*
Submit diagnostic test orders based on input from specific care providers. For each orderable item, the appropriate detail and instructions must be available for the ordering care provider to complete. Orders for diagnostic tests should be transmitted to the correct destination for completion or generate appropriate requisitions for communication to the relevant agencies.

☐ *Manage Order Sets (DC 1.4.3)*
Provide order sets based on provider input or system prompt. Order sets, which may include medication orders, allow a care provider to choose common orders for a particular circumstance or disease state according to best practice or other criteria. Recommended order sets may be presented based on patient data or other contexts.

☐ *Manage Referrals (DC 1.4.4)*
Enable the origination, documentation, and tracking of referrals between care providers or healthcare organizations, including clinical and administrative details of the referral. Documentation and tracking of a referral from one care provider to another is supported, whether the referred to or referring providers are internal or external to the healthcare organization. Guidelines for whether a particular referral for a particular patient is appropriate in a clinical context and with regard

to administrative factors such as insurance may be provided to the care provider at the time the referral is created.

☐ ***Manage Results (DC 1.4.5)***
Route, manage, and present current and historical test results to appropriate clinical personnel for review, with the ability to filter and compare results. Results of tests are presented in an easily accessible manner and to the appropriate care providers. Flow sheets, graphs, or other tools allow care providers to view or uncover trends in test data over time. In addition to making results viewable, it is often necessary to send results to appropriate care providers using an electronic messaging system, pager, or other mechanism. Results may also be routed to patients electronically or in the form of a letter.

☐ ***Order Blood Products and Other Biologics (DC 1.4.6)***
Communicate with appropriate sources or registries to order blood products or other biologics. Interact with a blood bank system or other source to manage orders for blood products or other biologics. Use of such products in the provision of care is captured. Blood bank or other functionality that may come under federal or other regulation (such as by the Food and Drug Administration [FDA] in the US) is not required; functional communication with such a system is required.

Consents, Authorizations, and Directives (DC 1.5)

☐ ***Manage Consents and Authorizations (DC 1.5.1)***
Create, maintain, and verify patient treatment decisions in the form of consents and authorizations when required. Treatment decisions are documented and include the extent of information, verification levels, and exposition of treatment options. This documentation helps ensure that decisions made at the discretion of the patient, family, or other responsible party govern the actual care that is delivered or withheld.

☐ ***Manage Patient Advance Directives (DC 1.5.2)***
Capture, maintain, and provide access to patient advance directives. Patient advance directives and provider do not resuscitate (DNR) orders can be captured. The date and circumstances under which the directives were received and the location of any paper records of advance directives can also be captured as appropriate.

Clinical Decision Support (DC 2.0)

Manage Health Information to Enable Decision Support (DC 2.1)

☐ ***Support of Standard Assessments (DC 2.1.1)***
Offer prompts to support the adherence to care plans, guidelines, and protocols at the point of information capture. When a clinician fills out an assessment, data entered triggers the system to prompt the assessor

to consider issues that would help assure a complete/accurate assessment. A simple demographic value or presenting problem (or combination) could provide a template for data gathering that represents best practice in this situation, eg, Type II diabetic review, fall and 70+, rectal bleeding, etc. As another example, to appropriately manage the use of restraints, an online alert is presented as defining the requirements for a behavioral health restraint when it is selected.

☐ *Support for Patient Context-Enabled Assessments (DC 2.1.2)*
Offer prompts based on patient-specific data at the point of information capture. When a clinician fills out an assessment, data entered are matched against data already in the system to identify potential linkages. For example, the system could span the medication list and the knowledge base to see if any of the symptoms are side effects of medication already prescribed. Important but rare diagnoses could be brought to the doctor's attention, for instance, ectopic pregnancy in a woman of child-bearing age who has abdominal pain.

☐ *Support for Identification of Potential Problems and Trends (DC 2.1.3)*
Identify trends that may lead to significant problems and provide prompts for consideration. When personal health information is collected directly during a patient visit that is input by the patient, or acquired from an external source (lab results), it is important to be able to identify potential problems and trends that may be patient specific, given the individual's personal health profile, or changes warranting further assessment. Examples include significant trends (eg, lab results, weight); decrease in creatinine clearance for a patient on metformin; or an abnormal increase in the international normalized ratio (INR) for a patient on warfarin.

☐ *Support for Patient and Family Preferences (DC 2.1.4)*
Support the integration of patient and family preferences into clinical decision support at all appropriate opportunities. Decision support functions should permit consideration of patient/family preference and concerns, such as with language, religion, culture, medication choice, invasive testing, and advance directives.

Care Plans, Guidelines, and Protocols (DC 2.2)

☐ *Support for Condition-Based Care Plans, Guidelines, and Protocols (DC 2.2.1)*

☐ **Support for Standard Care Plans, Guidelines, and Protocols (DC 2.2.1.1)**
Support the use of appropriate standard care plans, guidelines, and/or protocols for the management of specific conditions. At the

time of the clinical encounter, standard care protocols are presented. These may include site-specific considerations.

☐ **Support for Context-Sensitive Care Plans, Guidelines, and Protocols (DC 2.2.1.2)**

Identify and present the appropriate care plans, guidelines, and/or protocols for the management of specific conditions that are patient-specific. At the time of the clinical encounter (problem identification), recommendations for tests, treatments, medications, immunizations, referrals, and evaluations are presented based on evaluation of patient-specific data, the health profile, and any site-specific considerations. These may be modified on the basis of new clinical data at subsequent encounters.

☐ **Capture Variances from Standard Care Plans, Guidelines, and Protocols (DC 2.2.1.3)**

Identify variances from patient-specific and standard care plans, guidelines, and protocols. Variances from care plans, guidelines, or protocols are identified and tracked, with alerts, notifications, and reports as clinically appropriate. This may include systematic deviations from protocols or variances on a case-by-case basis dictated by the patient's particular circumstances.

☐ **Support Management of Patient Groups or Populations (DC 2.2.1.4)**

Provide support for the management of populations of patients that share diagnoses, problems, demographic characteristics, etc. Populations or groups of patients that share diagnoses (such as diabetes or hypertension), problems, demographic characteristics, and medication orders are identified. The clinician may be notified of eligibility for a particular test, therapy, or follow-up or may be notified of results from audits of compliance of these populations with disease management protocols.

☐ **Support for Research Protocols Relative to Individual Patient Care (DC 2.2.1.5)**

Provide support for the management of patients enrolled in research protocols and management of patients enrolled in research protocols. The clinician is presented with protocol-based care for patients enrolled in research studies. See *Enrollment of Patients (S 3.3.1)* for support for enrollment of patients in research protocols.

☐ **Support Self-Care (DC 2.2.1.6)**

Provide the patient with decision support for self-management of a condition between patient-provider encounters. Patients with specific conditions need to follow self-management plans that may include schedules for home monitoring, lab tests, and clinical check-ups; recommendations about nutrition, physical activity, tobacco use, etc; and guidance or reminders about medications.

Medication and Immunization Management (DC 2.3)

☐ *Support for Medications and Immunization Ordering (DC 2.3.1)*

☐ **Support for Drug Interaction Checking (DC 2.3.1.1)**
Identify drug interaction warnings at the point of medication ordering. The clinician is alerted to drug-drug, drug-allergy, and drug-food interactions at levels appropriate to the healthcare entity. These alerts may be customized to suit the user or group.

☐ **Patient-Specific Dosing and Warnings (DC 2.3.1.2)**
Identify and present appropriate dose recommendations based on patient-specific conditions and characteristics at the time of medication ordering. The clinician is alerted to drug condition interactions and patient-specific contraindications and warnings (eg, elite athlete, pregnancy, breast-feeding, and occupational risks). The preferences of the patient also may be presented (eg, reluctance to use an antibiotic). Additional patient parameters, including age, height, weight, [body surface area] BSA, may be incorporated.

☐ **Medication Recommendations (DC 2.3.1.3)**
Recommend treatment and monitoring on the basis of cost, local formularies, or therapeutic guidelines and protocols. Offer alternative treatments on the basis of best practice (eg, cost, adherence to guidelines), a generic brand, a different dosage, a different drug (watchful waiting). Suggest lab order monitoring as appropriate. Support expedited entry of series of medications that are part of a treatment regimen, such as renal dialysis, oncology, transplant medications, etc.

☐ *Support for Medication and Immunization Administration or Supply (DC 2.3.2)*
Alert providers in real time to potential administration errors such as wrong patient, wrong drug, wrong dose, wrong route, and wrong time in support of medication administration or pharmacy dispense/supply management and workflow. To reduce medication errors at the time of administration of a medication, the patient is positively identified; checks on the drug, the dose, the route, and the time are facilitated. Documentation is a by-product of this checking; administration details and additional patient information, such as injection site, vital signs, and pain assessments, are captured. In addition, access to online drug monograph information allows providers to check details about a drug and enhances patient education.

Orders, Referrals, Results, and Care Management (DC 2.4)

☐ *Support for Non-Medication Ordering (DC 2.4.1)*
Identify necessary order entry components for non-medication orders that make the order pertinent, relevant, and resource-conservative at

the time of provider order entry and flag any inappropriate orders based on patient profile. Possible order entry components include, but are not limited to: missing results required for the order, suggested corollary orders, notification of duplicate orders, institution-specific order guidelines, guideline-based orders/order sets, order sets, order reference text, and recommendations pertaining to the order that is specific to the patient diagnosis. Also, warnings for orders that may be inappropriate or contraindicated for specific patients (eg, x-rays for pregnant women) are presented.

☐ ***Support for Result Interpretation (DC 2.4.2)***
Evaluate results and notify provider of results within the context of the patient's clinical data. Possible result interpretations include, but are not limited to: abnormal result evaluation/notification, trending of results (eg, discrete lab values), evaluation of pertinent results at the time of provider order entry (eg, evaluation of lab results at the time of ordering a radiology exam), and evaluation of incoming results against active medication orders.

☐ ***Support for Referrals (DC 2.4.3)***

☐ **Support for Referral Process Based on Specific Patient's Clinical Data (DC 2.4.3.1)**
Evaluate referrals within the context of a patient's clinical data. When a healthcare referral is made, pertinent health information, including pertinent results, and demographic and insurance data elements (or lack thereof) are presented to the provider. Protocols for appropriate workup prior to referral may be presented.

☐ **Support for Referral Recommendations (DC 2.4.3.2)**
Evaluate patient data and recommend that a patient be referred based on the specific patient's clinical data. Entry of specific patient conditions may lead to recommendations for referral, such as for smoking cessation counseling if the patient is prescribed a medication to support cessation.

☐ ***Support for Care Delivery (DC 2.4.4)***

☐ **Support for Safe Blood Administration (DC 2.4.4.1)**
Alert provider in real time to potential blood administration errors. To reduce blood administration errors at the time of administration of blood products, the patient is positively identified and checks on the blood product, the amount, the route, and the time are facilitated. Documentation is a by-product of this checking.

☐ **Support for Accurate Specimen Collection (DC 2.4.4.2)**
Alert providers in real time to ensure specimen collection is supported. To ensure the accuracy of specimen collection, when a provider obtains specimens from a patient, the clinician can match each specimen collection identifier and the patient's ID bracelet. The provider is notified in real time of potential collection errors

such as wrong patient, wrong specimen type, wrong means of collection, wrong site, and wrong date and time. Documentation of the collection is a by-product of this checking.

Support of Health Maintenance: Preventive Care and Wellness (DC 2.5)

☐ **Present Alerts for Preventive Services and Wellness (DC 2.5.1)**
At the point of clinical decision making, identify patient-specific suggestions/reminders, screening tests/exams, and other preventive services in support of routine preventive and wellness patient care standards. At the time of an encounter, the provider or patient is presented with due or overdue activities based on protocols for preventive care and wellness. Examples include, but are not limited to, routine immunizations, adult and well baby care, and age- and sex-appropriate screening exams such as Pap smears.

☐ **Notifications and Reminders for Preventive Services and Wellness (DC 2.5.2)**
Between healthcare encounters, notify the patient and/or appropriate provider of those preventive services, tests, or behavioral actions that are due or overdue. The provider can generate notifications to patients regarding activities that are due or overdue, and these communications can be captured. Examples include, but are not limited to, time-sensitive patient and provider notification of follow-up appointments, laboratory tests, immunizations, and examinations. The notifications can be customized in terms of timing, repetitions, and administration reports. For example, a Pap test reminder might be sent to the patient two months prior to the test being due, repeated at three-month intervals, and then reported to the administrator or clinician when test is nine months overdue.

Support for Population Health (DC 2.6)

☐ **Support for Clinical Health State Monitoring Within a Population (DC 2.6.1)**
Support clinical health state monitoring of aggregate patient data for use in identifying health risks from the environment and/or population. Standardized surveillance performance measures that are based on known patterns of disease presentation can be identified by aggregating data from multiple input mechanisms. For example, elements include, but are not limited to, patient demographics, resource utilization, presenting symptoms, acute treatment regimens, laboratory and imaging study orders and results, and genomic and proteomic data elements. Identification of known patterns of existing diseases involves aggregation and analysis of these data elements by existing relationships. However, the

identification of new patterns of disease requires more sophisticated pattern recognition analysis. Early recognition of new patterns requires data points available early in the disease presentation. Demographics, ordering patterns, and resource use, such as ventilator or intensive care utilization pattern changes, are often available earlier in the presentation of non-predictable diseases. Consumer-generated information also is valuable with respect to surveillance efforts.

☐ ***Support for Notification and Response (DC 2.6.2)***
Upon notification by an external, authoritative source of a health risk within the cared-for population, alert relevant providers regarding specific, potentially at-risk patients with the appropriate level of notification. Upon receipt of notice of a health risk within a cared-for population from public health authorities or other external authoritative sources, identify and notify individual care providers or care managers that a risk has been identified and requires attention, including suggestions on the appropriate course of action. This process gives a care provider the ability to influence how patients are notified, if necessary.

☐ ***Support for Monitoring Response to Notifications (DC 2.6.3)***
In the event of a health risk alert and subsequent notification related to a specific patient, monitor if expected actions have been taken, and execute follow-up notification if they have not. Identifies that expected follow-up for a specific patient event, such as follow-up to error alerts or absence of an expected lab result, has not occurred, which calls for communication of the omission to appropriate care providers in the chain of authority. Of great importance to the notification process is the ability to match a care provider's clinical privileges with the clinical requirements of the notification.

Support for Knowledge Access (DC 2.7)

☐ ***Access Clinical Guidance (DC 2.7.1)***
Provide relevant evidence-based information and knowledge to the point of care for use in clinical decisions and care planning. Examples include, but are not limited to, evidence on treatment of conditions and wellness and context-specific links to other knowledge resources. When a condition is diagnosed, a provider is directed to relevant online evidence for management.

☐ ***Patient Knowledge Access (DC 2.7.2)***
Enable the accessibility of reliable information about wellness, disease management, treatments, and related information that is relevant for a specific patient. An individual will be able to find reliable information to answer a health question, follow-up from a clinical visit, identify treatment options, or other health information needs. The information may be linked directly from entries in the health record or may be accessed through other means such as key word searching.

Operations Management and Communication (DC 3.0)

☐ **Clinical Workflow Tasking (DC 3.1)**

Schedule and manage tasks with appropriate timeliness. Since the electronic health record (EHR) will replace the paper chart, tasks that were based on the paper artifact must be effectively managed in the electronic environment. Functions must exist in the electronic health record system that electronically support any workflow that previously depended on the existence of a physical artifact in a paper-based system, such as a paper chart or a phone message slip. Tasks differ from other more generic communication among participants in the care process because they are a call to action and target completion of a specific workflow in the context of a patient's health record, including a specific component of the record. Tasks also require disposition (final resolution). The initiator may optionally require a response. For example, in a paper-based system, physically placing charts in piles for review creates a physical queue of tasks related to those charts. This queue of tasks, such as a set of patient phone calls to be returned, must be supported electronically so that the list of patients to be called is visible to the appropriate user or role for disposition. Tasks are time limited or finite. The state transition—created, performed, and resolved—may be managed by the user explicitly or automatically based on rules. For example, if a user has a task to sign off on a test result, that task should automatically be marked complete by the EHR when the test result lined to the task is signed in the system. Patients will become more involved in the care process by receiving tasks related to their care. Examples of patient-related tasks include acknowledgment of receipt of test result forwarded from the provider or a request to schedule an appointment for a Pap smear (based on age and frequency criteria) generated automatically by the electronic health record system on behalf of the provider.

☐ *Clinical Task Assignment and Routing (DC 3.1.1)*

Assignment, delegation, and/or transmission of tasks to the appropriate parties. Tasks are at all times assigned to at least one user or role for disposition. Whether the task is assignable and to whom the task can be assigned will be determined by the specific needs of practitioners in a care setting. Task-assignment lists help users prioritize and complete assigned tasks. For example, after receiving a phone call from a patient, the triage nurse routes or assigns a task to return the patient's call to the physician who is on call. Task creation and assignment may be automated, where appropriate. An example of a system-triggered task is when lab results are received electronically: a task to review the result is automatically generated and assigned to a clinician. Task assignment ensures that all tasks are disposed of by the appropriate person or role and allows efficient interaction of entities in the care process.

☐ *Clinical Task Linking (DC 3.1.2)*
Linkage of tasks to patients and/or a relevant part of the electronic health record. Clinical tasks are linked to patient or to a component of a patient's medical record. An example of a well-defined task is: "Dr Jones must review Mr Smith's blood work results." Efficient workflow is facilitated by navigating to the appropriate area of the record to ensure that the appropriate test result for the correct patient is reviewed. Other examples of tasks might involve fulfillment of orders or responding to patient phone calls.

☐ *Clinical Task Tracking (DC 3.1.3)*
Track tasks to guarantee that each task is carried out and completed appropriately. In order to reduce the risk of errors during the care process due to missed tasks, the provider is able to view and track non-disposed tasks, current work lists, the status of each task, unassigned tasks, or other tasks where a risk of omission exists. For example, a provider is able to create a report to show test results that have not been reviewed by the ordering provider based on an interval appropriate to the care setting.

☐ **Clinical Task Timeliness Tracking (DC 3.1.3.1)**
Track and/or report on timeliness of task completion. Capability to track and review reports on the timeliness of certain tasks in accordance with relevant law and accreditation standards.

☐ **Support Clinical Communication (DC 3.2)**
Healthcare requires secure communications among various participants: patients, doctors, nurses, chronic disease care managers, pharmacies, laboratories, payers, consultants, etc. An effective electronic health record system supports communication across all relevant participants, reduces the overhead and costs of healthcare-related communications, and provides automatic tracking and reporting. The list of communication participants is determined by the care setting and may change over time. Because of concerns about scalability of the specification over time, communication participants for all care settings or across care settings are not enumerated here because it would limit the possibilities available to each care setting and implementation. However, communication between providers and between patients and providers will be supported in all appropriate care settings and across care settings. Implementation of the electronic health record system enables new and more effective channels of communication, significantly improving efficiency and patient care. **The communication functions of the electronic health record system will eventually change the way participants collaborate and distribute the work of patient care.** [Emphasis added by authors.]

☐ *Inter-Provider Communication (DC 3.2.1)*

Support secure inbound and outbound electronic communication between providers to trigger or respond to pertinent actions in the care process, including referral; document non-electronic communication, such as phone calls, correspondence, or other encounters; and generate paper message artifacts, where appropriate. Communication among providers involved in the care process can range from real-time communication, such as fulfillment of an injection while the patient is in the exam room, to asynchronous communication, such as consultation reports between physicians. Some forms of inter-practitioner communication will be paper based and the electronic health record system must be able to produce appropriate documents.

☐ *Pharmacy Communication (DC 3.2.2)*

Provide features to enable secure bidirectional communication of information electronically between practitioners and pharmacies or between practitioner and intended recipient of pharmacy orders. This communication is used when a medication is prescribed and routed to the pharmacy or another intended recipient of pharmacy orders. This information is used to avoid transcription errors and facilitate detection of potential adverse reactions. Upon filling the prescription, information is sent back to the practitioner to indicate that the patient received the medication. If there is a question from the pharmacy, that communication can be presented to the provider with other tasks.

☐ *Provider and Patient or Family Communication (DC 3.2.3)*

Trigger or respond to inbound and outbound electronic communication between providers and patients or patient representatives with pertinent actions in the care process. The clinician is able to communicate with patients and others, capturing the nature and content of electronic communication or the time and details of other communication. Examples include when test results arrive, the clinician may wish to send an e-mail the patient that the test results were normal (details of this communication are captured); a patient may wish to request a refill of medication by sending an e-mail message to the physician; patients with asthma may wish to communicate their peak flow logs/diaries to their providers; and a hospital may wish to communicate with selected patients about a new smoking cessation program.

☐ *Patient, Family, and Caregiver Education (DC 3.2.4)*

Identify and make available electronically or in print any educational or support resources for patients, families, and caregivers that are most pertinent for a given health concern, condition, or diagnosis and appropriate for the person(s). The provider or patient is presented with a library of educational materials and, where appropriate, given the opportunity to document patient/caregiver comprehension. The materials can be printed or electronically communicated to the patient.

☐ ***Communication With Medical Devices (DC 3.2.5)***
Support communication and presentation of data captured from medical devices. Communication with medical devices is supported as appropriate to the care setting. Examples include vital signs/ pulse oximeter; anesthesia machines; home diagnostic devices for chronic disease management; laboratory machines; and bar-coded artifacts, such as medicine, immunizations, demographics, history, and identification.

SUPPORTIVE

Clinical Support (S 1.0)

☐ **Registry Notification (S 1.1)**
Enable the automated transfer of formatted demographic and clinical information to and from local disease-specific registries and other notifiable registries for patient monitoring and subsequent epidemiological analysis. The user can export personal health information to disease-specific registries and other notifiable registries like immunization registries and add new registries through the addition of standard data transfer protocols or messages.

☐ **Donor Management Support (S 1.2)**
Provide capability to capture or receive and share needed information on potential organ and blood donors and recipients. The user is able to capture or receive information on potential organ and blood donors and recipients. The user can make this information available to internal and external donor-matching agencies.

☐ **Provider Directory (S 1.3)**
Provide a current directory of practitioner, team, department, organization, etc, information in accordance with relevant laws, regulations, and conventions. Maintain or access current directory of provider information in accordance with relevant laws, regulations, and conventions, including full name, address, or physical location, as well as a 24/7 telecommunications address, such as telephone or pager access number, for purposes of the following functions:

☐ ***Provider Demographics (S 1.3.1)*** ˙
Provide a current directory of practitioners that, in addition to demographic information, contains data needed to determine levels of access required by the EHR security system. Provider demographics

may include any credentials, certifications, or any other information that may be used to verify that a provider is permitted to perform certain services.

☐ ***Provider's Location Within Facility (S 1.3.2)***
Provide provider location or contact information on a facility's premises.

☐ ***Provider's On-Call Location (S 1.3.3)***
Provide provider location or contact information when on call.

☐ ***Provider's General Location (S 1.3.4)***
Provide locations or contact information for the provider in order to direct patients or queries.

☐ **Patient Directory (S 1.4)**
Provide a current directory of patient information in accordance with relevant privacy and other applicable laws, regulations, and conventions. Provide a current directory of patient information in accordance with relevant privacy and other applicable laws, regulations, and conventions, including, when available, full name, address or physical location, alternate contact person, primary phone number, and relevant health status information for the purposes of the following functions:

☐ ***Patient Demographics (S 1.4.1)***
Support interactions with other systems, applications, and modules to enable the maintenance of updated demographic information in accordance with realm-specific record-keeping requirements. The minimum demographic data set must include the data required by realm-specific laws governing healthcare transactions and reporting. This also may include data input of death status information.

☐ ***Patient's Location Within a Facility (S 1.4.2)***
Provide the patient's location information within a facility's premises. An example is the patient census in a hospital setting.

☐ ***Patient's Residence for the Provision and Administration of Services (S 1.4.3)***
Provide the patient's residence information solely for purposes related to the provision and administration of services to the patient, patient transport, and as required for public health reporting.

☐ ***Optimize Patient Bed Assignment (S 1.4.4)***
Support interactions with other systems, applications, and modules to ensure that the patient's bed assignments within the facility optimize care and minimize risks, such as exposure to contagious patients.

☐ **De-Identified Data Request Management (S 1.5)**
Provide patient data in a manner that meets local requirements for de-identification. When an internal or external party requests patient data and that party requests de-identified data, or is not entitled to identify

patient information, either by law or custom, the user can export the data in a fashion that meets local requirements for de-identification. An audit trail of these requests and exports is maintained. For internal clinical audit, a re-identification key may be added to the data.

☐ **Scheduling (S 1.6)**

Support interactions with other systems, applications, and modules to provide the necessary data to a scheduling system for optimal efficiency in the scheduling of patient care, for either the patient or a resource/ device. The system's user can schedule events as required. Relevant clinical or demographic information can be linked to the task.

☐ **Healthcare Resource Availability (S 1.7)**

Support interactions with other systems, applications, and modules to enable the distribution of local healthcare resource information in times of local or national emergencies. In times of identified local or national emergencies and upon request from authorized bodies, provide current status of health resources, including, but not limited to, available beds, providers, support personnel, ancillary care areas and devices, operating theaters, medical supplies, vaccines, and pharmaceuticals. The intent is for the authorized body to distribute either resources or patient load to maximize efficient healthcare delivery.

Measurement, Analysis, Research, and Reports (S 2.0)

☐ **Measurement, Monitoring, and Analysis (S 2.1)**

Support measurement and monitoring of care for relevant purposes.

☐ *Outcome Measures and Analysis (S 2.1.1)*

Support the capture and reporting of information for the analysis of outcomes of care provided to populations, in facilities, by providers, and in communities.

☐ *Performance and Accountability Measures (S 2.1.2)*

Support the capture and reporting of quality, performance, and accountability measures to which providers/facilities/delivery systems/ communities are held accountable, including measures related to process, outcomes, and costs of care, and which may be used in "pay for performance" monitoring and adherence to best practice guidelines.

☐ **Report Generation (S 2.2)**

Provide report generation features for the generation of standard and ad hoc reports. A user can create standard and ad hoc reports for clinical, administrative, and financial decision-making, and for patient use, including structured data and unstructured text from the patient's health record. Reports may be linked with financial and other external data sources that have data external to the entity. Such reports may include patient level reports, provider/facility/delivery system level reports, population level reports, and reports to public health agencies. Examples are:

1. Patient level reports include administratively required patient assessment forms, admission/transfer/discharge reports, operative and procedure reports, consultation reports, and drug profiles.

2. Population level reports include reports on the effectiveness of clinical pathways and other evidence-based practices, tracking completeness of clinical documentation, etc.

3. Reports to public health agencies include vital statistics, reportable diseases, discharge summaries, immunization data with adverse outcomes, cancer data, other such data necessary to maintain public health, and suspicions of newly emerging infectious disease and nonnatural events.

☐ ***Health Record Output (S 2.2.1)***
Allow users to define the records and reports that are considered the formal health record for disclosure purposes and provide a mechanism for both chronological and specified record element output. Provide hard copy and electronic output that can fully chronicle the healthcare process, support selection of specific sections of the health record, and allow healthcare organizations to define the report and documents that will comprise the formal health record for disclosure purposes.

Administrative and Financial (S 3.0)

☐ **Encounter/Episode of Care Management (S 3.1)**
Manage and document the healthcare needed and delivered during an encounter/episode of care. Using data standards and technologies that support interoperability, encounter management promotes patient centered/oriented care and enables real-time, immediate point-of-service/point-of-care by facilitating efficient workflow and operations performance to ensure the integrity of

1. The health record.
2. Public health, financial, and administrative reporting.
3. The healthcare delivery process.

This support is necessary for direct care functionality that relies on providing user interaction and workflows, which are configured according to clinical protocols and business rules based on encounter-specific values, such as care setting, inpatient, outpatient, home health, and other encounter types, provider type, patient's EHR, health status, demographics, and the initial purpose of the encounter.

☐ *Specialized Views (S 3.1.1)*
Present specialized views based on encounter-specific values, clinical protocols, and business rules. The system user is presented with a presentation view and system interaction appropriate to the context with capture of encounter-specific values, clinical protocols, and business rules. This "user view" may be configurable by the user or system technicians. For example, a mobile home healthcare worker using a wireless laptop at a patient's home would be presented with a home healthcare workflow that is synchronized to the current patient's care plan and tailored to support the interventions appropriate for this patient, including chronic disease management protocols.

☐ *Encounter-Specific Functionality (S 3.1.2)*
Provide assistance in assembling appropriate data, supporting data collection, and processing output from a specific encounter. Workflows, based on encounter management settings, will assist in determining the appropriate data collection, import, export, extraction, linkages, and transformation. For example, a pediatrician is presented with diagnostic and procedure codes specific to pediatrics. Business rules enable automatic collection of necessary data from the patient's health record and patient registry. As the provider enters data, workflow processes are triggered to populate appropriate transactions and documents, such as an eligibility verification transaction or query of the immunization registry.

☐ *Automatic Generation of Administrative and Financial Data From Clinical Record (S 3.1.3)*
Provide patients clinical data to support administrative and financial reporting. A user can generate a bill based on health record data. Maximizing the extent to which administrative and financial data can be derived or developed from clinical data will lessen provider reporting burdens and the time it takes to complete administrative and financial processes, such as claim reimbursement. This may be implemented by mapping of clinical terminologies in use to administrative and financial terminologies.

☐ *Support Remote Healthcare Services (S 3.1.4)*
Support remote healthcare services, such as telehealth and remote device monitoring, by integrating records and data collected by these means into the patient's EHR for care management, billing, and public health purposes. Enable remote treatment of patients using monitoring devices and two-way communications between provider and patient or provider and provider. Promote patient empowerment, self-determination, and ability to maintain health status in the community. Promote personal health, wellness, and preventive care. For example, a diabetic pregnant mother can

self-monitor her condition from her home, use Web TV to report to her provider, and get dietary and other health promoting information to assist her with managing her high-risk pregnancy.

☐ **Information Access for Supplemental Use (S 3.2)**
Support extraction, transformation, and linkage of information from structured data and unstructured text in the patient's health record for care management and financial, administrative, and public health purposes. Using data standards and technologies that support interoperability, information access functionalities serve primary and secondary record use and reporting with continuous record availability and access that ensure the integrity of:

1. The health record
2. Public health, financial, and administrative reporting
3. The healthcare delivery process.

☐ *Rules-Driven Clinical Coding Assistance (S 3.2.1)*
Make available all pertinent patient information needed to support coding of diagnoses, procedures, and outcomes. The user is assisted in coding information for clinical reporting reasons. For example, a professional coder may have to code the principal diagnosis in the current, applicable International Classification of Diseases (ICD) as a basis for hospital funding. All diagnoses and procedures during the episode may be presented to the coder, as well as the applicable ICD hierarchy containing these codes.

☐ *Rules-Driven Financial and Administrative Coding Assistance (S 3.2.2)*
Provide financial and administrative coding assistance based on structured data and unstructured text available in the encounter documentation. The user is assisted in coding information for billing or administrative reasons. For example, the Health Insurance Portability and Accountability Act of 1996 (HIPAA) 837 Professional Claim requires the date of the last menstrual cycle for claims involving pregnancy. To support the generation of this transaction, the clinician would need to be prompted to enter this date when the patient is first determined to be pregnant, thereby making this information available for the billing process.

☐ *Integrate Cost/Financial Information (S 3.2.3)*
Support interactions with other systems, applications, and modules to enable the use of cost management information required to guide users and workflows. The provider is alerted or presented with the most cost-effective services, referrals, devices, etc, to recommend to the patient. This may be tailored to the patient's health insurance/plan coverage rules. Medications may be presented in order of cost or the cost of specific interventions may be presented at the time of ordering.

☐ **Administrative Transaction Processing (S 3.3)**

Support the creation, using external data sources, if necessary, of electronic interchange and processing of transactions that may be necessary for encounter management during an episode of care. Electronic health record systems (EHR-S) support the creation, using external data sources, if necessary, of electronic interchange and processing of transactions that follow that may be necessary for encounter management during an episode of care. The EHR-S:

1. Captures the patient health-related information needed for administrative and financial purposes, including reimbursement.

2. Captures episode and encounter information to pass to administrative or financial processes, which triggers transmissions of charge transactions as a by-product of online interaction, including order entry, order status, result entry, documentation entry, and medication administration charting.

3. Automatically retrieves information needed to verify coverage and medical necessity.

4. Captures and presents all patient information needed to support coding, as a by-product of care delivery and documentation. Ideally, coding is performed based on documentation.

5. Reduces denials and error rates in claims as part of the clinically automated revenue cycle.

6. Provides clinical information availability needed for billing on date of service.

7. Eliminates physician and clinical teams performing additional data entry/tasks exclusively to support administrative or financial processes.

☐ *Enrollment of Patients (S 3.3.1)*

Support interactions with other systems, applications, and modules to enable enrollment of uninsured patients into subsidized and unsubsidized health plans and enrollment of patients who are eligible on the basis of health and financial status in social service and other programs, including clinical trials. Enrollment expedites determination of health insurance coverage, thereby increasing patient access to care. The provider may be alerted that uninsured patients may be eligible for subsidized health insurance or other health programs because they meet eligibility criteria based on demographics or health status. For example, a provider is notified that the uninsured parents of a child enrolled in a State Children's Health Insurance Program (S-CHIP) may now be eligible for a new subsidized health insurance program. As another example, a provider presents a recently immigrated pregnant patient with information about eligibility for subsidy. Links may be provided to online enrollment forms. When enrollment is determined, health coverage information needed for processing administrative and financial documentation, reports, and transactions is captured.

☐ ***Eligibility Verification and Determination of Coverage (S 3.3.2)***
Support interactions with other systems, applications, and modules to enable eligibility verification for health insurance and special programs, including verification of benefits and predetermination of coverage. Automatically retrieves information needed to support verification of coverage at the appropriate point in the encounter workflow. Improves patient access to covered care and reduces claim denials. When eligibility is verified, the EHR-S would capture eligibility information needed for processing administrative and financial documentation, reports, and transactions and would update or flag any inconsistent data. In addition to health insurance eligibility, this function would support verification of registration in programs and registries, such as chronic care case management and immunization registries. The EHR-S likely would verify health insurance eligibility prior to the encounter, but would verify registration in case management or immunization registries during the encounter.

☐ ***Service Authorizations (S 3.3.3)***
Support interactions with other systems, applications, and modules to enable the creation of request, response, and appeals related to service authorization, including prior authorizations, referrals, and pre-certification. Automatically retrieves information needed to support verification of medical necessity and prior authorization of services at the appropriate point in the encounter workflow. Improves timeliness of patient care and reduces claim denials.

☐ ***Support of Service Requests and Claims (S 3.3.4)***
Support interactions with other systems, applications, and modules to support the creation of healthcare attachments for submitting additional clinical information in support of service requests and claims. Automatically retrieves structured data, including lab, imaging, and device monitoring data, and unstructured text based on rules or requests for additional clinical information in support of service requests or claims at the appropriate point in the encounter workflow.

☐ ***Claims and Encounter Reports for Reimbursement (S 3.3.5)***
Support interactions with other systems, applications, and modules to enable the creation of claims and encounter reports for

reimbursement. Automatically retrieves information needed to support claims and encounter reporting at the appropriate point in the encounter workflow.

☐ ***Health Service Reports at the Conclusion of an Episode of Care (S 3.3.6)***
Support the creation of health service reports at the conclusion of an episode of care. Support the creation of health service reports to authorized health entities, such as public health authorities. Examples that a provider may be required to generate at the conclusion of an episode of care are notifiable condition reports containing immunization, cancer registry, and discharge data. Effective use of this function means that clinicians do not perform additional data entry to support health management programs and reporting.

☐ **Manage Practitioner/Patient Relationships (S 3.4)**
Identify relationships among providers treating a single patient and provide the ability to manage patient lists assigned to a particular provider. This function addresses the ability to access and update current information about the relationships between caregivers and the subjects of care. This information should be able to flow seamlessly between the different components of the EHR-S and between the EHR-S and other systems. Business rules may be reflected in the presentation of and access to this information. The relationship among providers treating a single patient will include any necessary chain of authority/responsibility. Examples of this function are:

1. In a care setting with multiple providers in which the patient can only see certain kinds of providers or an individual provider, allows the selection of only the appropriate providers.

2. The user is presented with a list of people assigned to a given practitioner and may alter the assignment as required to a group or to another individual or by sharing the assignment.

☐ **Subject-to-Subject Relationship (S 3.5)**
Capture relationships between patients and others to facilitate appropriate access to a health record on a relationship basis, such as a parental access of a child's health record. A user may assign the relationship of parent to a person who is an offspring of the parent. This relationship may facilitate access by the parent to the health record of a child.

☐ ***Related by Genealogy (S 3.5.1)***
Provide information of Related by Genealogy: blood relatives.

☐ ***Related by Insurance (S 3.5.2)***
Support interactions with other systems, applications, and modules to provide information of Related by Insurance: domestic partner, spouse, and guarantor.

☐ ***Related by Living Situation (S 3.5.3)***
Provide information of Related by Living Situation: in the same household.

☐ ***Related by Other Means (S 3.5.4)***
Provide information of Related by Other Means: epidemiologic exposure or other person authorized to see records, such as in living will cases.

☐ **Acuity and Severity (S 3.6)**
Provide the data necessary for the capability to support and manage patient acuity/severity of illness/risk adjustment.

☐ **Maintenance of Supportive Functions (S 3.7)**
Update EHR supportive content on an automated basis.

☐ ***Clinical Decision Support System Guidelines Updates (S 3.7.1)***
Receive and validate formatted inbound communications to facilitate updating of clinical decision support system guidelines and associated reference material.

☐ ***Account for Patient Education Material Updates (S 3.7.2)***
Receive and validate formatted inbound communications to facilitate updating of patient education material.

☐ ***Patient Reminder Information Updates (S 3.7.3)***
Receive and validate formatted inbound communications to facilitate updating of patient reminder information from external sources such as cancer or immunization registries.

☐ ***Public Health-Related Updates (S 3.7.4)***
Receive and validate formatted inbound communications to facilitate updating of public health reporting guidelines.

INFORMATION INFRASTRUCTURE

Electronic Health Record Security (I 1.0)

Secure access to an electronic health records system (EHR-S) and electronic health record (EHR) information. Manage the sets of access control permissions granted within an EHR-S. Prevent unauthorized use of data, data loss, tampering, and destruction. To enforce security, all EHR-S applications must adhere to the rules established to control access and protect the privacy of EHR information. Security measures assist in preventing unauthorized use of data and protect against loss, tampering, and destruction.

☐ **Entity Authentication (I 1.1)**
Authenticate EHR-S users and/or entities before allowing access to an EHR-S. Both users and application are subject to authentication.

The EHR-S must provide mechanisms for users and applications to be authenticated. Users will have to be authenticated when they attempt to use the application. The applications must authenticate themselves before accessing EHR information managed by other applications or remote EHR-Ss. In order for authentication to be established, a chain-of-trust agreement is assumed to be in place. Examples of entity authentication include:

☐ Username/password

☐ Digital certificate

☐ Secure token

☐ Biometrics.

☐ **Entity Authorization (I 1.2)**
Manage the sets of access-control permissions granted to entities that use an EHR-S (EHR-S users). Enable EHR-S security administrators to grant authorizations to users, for roles, and within contexts. A combination of the authorization levels may be applied to control access to EHR-S functions or data within an EHR-S, including at the application or the operating system level. Entities that use an EHR-S (EHR-S users) are authorized to use the components of an EHR-S according to identity, role, work assignment, present condition, and/or location in accordance with an entity's scope of practice within a legal jurisdiction.

☐ *User-based authorization* refers to the permissions granted or denied based on the identity of an individual. An example of user-based authorization is a patient-defined denial of access to all or part of a record to a particular party for reasons such as privacy. Another example is user-based authorization for a telemonitor device or robotic access to an EHR-S for prescribed directions and other input.

☐ *Role-based authorization* refers to the responsibility or function performed in a particular operation or process. Examples include an application or device, such as a telemonitor or robotic, and a nurse, dietician, administrator, legal guardian, or auditor.

☐ *Context-based authorization* is defined by the International Organization for Standardization (ISO) as security-relevant properties of the context in which an access request occurs, explicitly: time, location, route of access, and quality of authentication. For example, an EHR-S might only allow supervising providers' context authorization to attest to entries proposed by residents under their supervision. In addition to the standard, context authorization for an EHR-S is extended to satisfy special circumstances such as assignment, consents, or other factors related to healthcare. A context-based example might be a right granted for a limited period to view those, and only those, EHR records connected to a specific topic of investigation.

☐ **Entity Access Control (I 1.3)**

Verify and enforce access control to all EHR-S components, EHR information, and functions for end users, applications, sites, etc, to prevent unauthorized use of a resource, including the prevention or use of a resource in an unauthorized manner. This is a fundamental function of an EHR-S. To ensure access is controlled, an EHR-S must perform an identity lookup of users or application for any operation that requires it (authentication, authorization, secure routing, querying, etc) and enforce the system and information access rules that have been defined.

☐ *Patient Access Management (I 1.3.1)*

Enable a healthcare professional to manage a patient's access to the patient's personal health information. Patient access management includes allowing a patient access to the patient's information and restricting access by the patient or guardian to information that is potentially harmful to the patient. A healthcare professional will be able to manage a patient's ability to view his/her EHR and to alert other providers accessing the EHR about any constraints on patient access placed by this provider. Typically, a patient has the right to view his/her EHR. However, a healthcare provider may sometimes need to prevent a patient or guardian from viewing parts of the record. For example, a patient receiving psychiatric care might harm himself (or others) if he reads the doctor's evaluation of his condition. Furthermore, reading the doctor's therapy plan might actually cause the plan to fail.

☐ **Non-Repudiation (I 1.4)**

Limit an EHR-S user's ability to deny (repudiate) an electronic data exchange originated, received, or authorized by that user. Non-repudiation ensures that an entered or transferred message has been entered, sent, or received by the parties claiming to have entered, sent, or received the message. Non-repudiation is a way to guarantee that the sender of a message cannot later deny having sent the message and that the recipient cannot deny having received the message. Non-repudiation may be achieved through the use of:

☐ Digital signature, which serves as a unique identifier for an individual, much like a written signature.

☐ Confirmation service, which utilizes a message transfer agent to create a digital receipt, providing confirmation that a message was sent and/or received.

☐ Timestamp, which proves that a document existed at a certain date and time.

☐ **Secure Data Exchange (I 1.5)**

Secure all modes of EHR data exchange. Whenever an exchange of EHR information occurs, it requires appropriate security and privacy considerations, including data obfuscation and destination and source authentication, when necessary. For example, it may be necessary to encrypt data sent to remote or external destinations. This function requires that there is an overall coordination regarding what information is exchanged between EHR-S entities and how that exchange is expected to occur. The policies applied at different locations must be consistent or compatible with each other in order to ensure that the information is protected when it crosses entity boundaries within an EHR-S or external to an EHR-S.

☐ **Secure Data Routing (I 1.6)**

Route electronically exchanged EHR data only to/from known, registered, and authenticated destinations/sources, according to applicable healthcare-specific rules and relevant standards. An EHR-S needs to ensure that it is exchanging EHR information with the entities (applications, institutions, and directories) that it expects. This function depends on entity authorization and authentication to be available in the system. For example, a physician practice management application in an EHR-S might send claim attachment information to an external entity. To accomplish this, the application must use a secure routing method, which ensures that both the sender and receiving side are authorized to engage in the information exchange.

☐ **Information Attestation (I 1.7)**

Manage electronic attestation of information including the retention of the signature of attestation (or certificate of authenticity) associated with incoming or outgoing information. The purpose of attestation is to show authorship and assign responsibility for an act, event, condition, opinion, or diagnosis. Every entity in the health record must be identified with the author and should not be made or signed by someone other than the author. A transcriptionist may transcribe an author's notes and a senior clinician may attest to the accuracy of another's statement of events. Attestation is required for paper or electronic entries such as narrative or progress notes, assessments, flow sheets, and orders. Digital signatures may be used to implement document attestation. For an incoming document, the record of attestation is retained, if included. Attestation functionality must meet applicable legal, regulatory, and other applicable standards or requirements.

☐ **Enforcement of Confidentiality (I 1.8)**

Enforce the applicable jurisdiction's patient privacy rules as they apply to various parts of an EHR-S through the implementation of security mechanisms. A patient's privacy may be adversely affected when EHRs are not held in confidence. Privacy rule enforcement decreases unauthorized access and promotes the level of EHR confidentiality.

Electronic Health Record Information and Records Management (I 2.0)

☐ **Data Retention, Availability, and Destruction (I 2.1)**
Retain, ensure availability, and destroy health record information according to organizational standards. This includes:

☐ *Retaining all EHR-S data and clinical documents for the time period designated by policy or legal requirement.*

☐ *Retaining inbound documents as originally received (unaltered).*

☐ *Ensuring availability of information for the legally prescribed period of time.*

☐ *Providing ability to destroy EHR data/records in a systematic way according to policy and after the legally prescribed retention period.*

Discrete and structured EHR-S data, records, and reports must be:

☐ Made available to users in a timely fashion.

☐ Stored and retrieved in a semantically intelligent and useful manner, such as chronologically, retrospectively per a given disease or event, or in accordance with business requirements, local policies, or legal requirements.

☐ Retained for a legally defined period of time.

☐ Destroyed in a systematic manner in relation to the applicable retention period.

An EHR-S also must allow an organization to identify data/records to be destroyed and to review and approve destruction before it occurs.

☐ **Audit Trail (I 2.2)**
Provide audit trail capabilities for resource access and usage indicating the author, the modification, where pertinent, and the data and time at which a record was created, modified, viewed, extracted, or deleted. Audit trails extend to information exchange and to audit of consent status management[9] and to entity authentication attempts. Audit functionality includes the ability to generate audit reports and to interactively view change history for individual health records or for an EHR-S. Audit functionality extends to security audits, data audits, audits of data exchange, and the ability to generate audit reports. Audit trail settings should be configurable to meet the needs of local policies. Examples of audited areas include:

☐ Security audit, which logs access attempts and resource usage, including user login, file access, and other activities and whether any actual or attempted security violations occurred.

☐ Data audit, which records who, when, and by which system an EHR record was created, updated, translated, viewed, extracted, or, if local policy permits, deleted. Audit data may refer to system setup data or to clinical patient management data.

☐ Information exchange audit, which records data exchanged between EHR-S applications, such as sending application; the nature, history, and content of information exchanged; and information about data transformations, like vocabulary translations, reception event details, etc.

☐ Audit reports should be flexible and address users' needs. For example, a legal authority may want to know how many patients a given healthcare provider treated while the provider's license was suspended. As another example, a report detailing all persons who modified or viewed a certain patient record may be needed.

☐ Security audit trails and data audit trails are used to verify enforcement of business, data integrity, security, and access-control rules.

There is a requirement for system audit trails for the following events:

☐ Loading new versions of, making changes to, the clinical system.
☐ Loading new versions of codes and knowledge bases.
☐ Changing the date and time where the clinical system allows this to be done.
☐ Taking and restoring of backup.
☐ Archiving any data.
☐ Reactivating an archived patient record.
☐ Entry to and exiting from the clinical system.
☐ Connecting via remote access, including such connections for system support and maintenance activities.

☐ **Synchronization (I 2.3)**
Maintain synchronization involving:
☐ Interaction with entity directories.
☐ Linkage of received data with existing entity records.
☐ Location of each health record component.
☐ Communication of changes between key systems.

An EHR-S may consist of a set of components or applications, where each application manages a subset of the health information. Therefore, it is important that, through interoperability mechanisms, an EHR-S maintains all the relevant information regarding the health record in synchrony. For example, if a physician orders an MRI, a set of diagnostic images and a radiology report will be created. The patient demographics, the order for the MRI, the diagnostic images associated with the order, and the report associated with the study must all be synchronized in order for the clinicians to view the complete record.

☐   **Extraction of Health Record Information (I 2.4)**
Manage data extraction in accordance with analysis and reporting requirements. The extracted data may require use of more than one application and it may be pre-processed before transmission, such as being de-identified. Data extractions may be used to exchange data and provide reports for primary and ancillary purposes. An EHR-S enables an authorized user, such as a clinician, to access and aggregate the distributed information, which corresponds to the health record or records that are needed for viewing, reporting, disclosure, etc. An EHR-S must support data extraction operations across the complete data set that constitutes the health record of an individual and provide an output that fully chronicles the healthcare process. Data extractions are used as input to continuity of care records. In addition, data extractions can be used for administrative, financial, research, quality analysis, and public health purposes.

Unique Identity, Registry, and Directory Services (I 3.0)

☐   **Distributed Registry Access (I 3.1)**
Enable system communication with registry services through standardized interfaces and extend to services provided externally to an EHR-S. An EHR-S relies on a set of infrastructure services, directories, and registries, which may be organized hierarchically or federated, that support communication between EHR-Ss. For example, a patient treated by a primary care physician for a chronic condition may become ill while out of town. The new provider's EHR-S interrogates a local, regional, or national registry to find the patient's previous records. From the primary care record, a remote EHR-S retrieves relevant information in conformance with applicable patient privacy and confidentiality rules. An example of local registry usage is an EHR-S application sending a query message to the Hospital Information System to retrieve a patient's demographic data.

Health Informatics and Terminology Standards (I 4.0)

Ensure consistent terminologies, data correctness, and interoperability in accordance with realm-specific requirements by complying with standards for healthcare transactions, vocabularies, code sets, and artifacts, such as templates, system interfaces, decision-support syntax and algorithms, and clinical document architecture. Support reference to standard and local terminologies and their versions in a manner that ensures comparable and consistent use of vocabulary, such as the Common Terminology Services specification. Examples that an EHR-S needs to support are a consistent set of terminologies such as Logical Observation Identifiers Names and Codes (LOINC), Systematized Nomenclature of Medicine-Clinical Terms (SNOMED-CT), applicable ICD, and Current Procedural Terminology (CPT®),[10] and messaging standards, such as X12[11] and HL7. Vocabularies may be provided through a terminology service internal or external to an EHR-S.

☐ **Maintenance and Versioning of Health Informatics and Terminology Standards (I 4.1)**
Enable version control according to customized policies to ensure maintenance of utilized standards. Version control allows for multiple sets or versions of the same terminology to exist and be distinctly recognized over time. Terminology versioning supports retrospective analysis and research and interoperability with systems that comply with different releases of the standard. Similar functionality must exist for messaging and other informatics-based standards. It should be possible to retire depreciated versions when applicable business cycles are completed while maintaining obsolescent code sets for possible claims adjustment throughout a claim's life cycle.

☐ **Mapping Local Terminology, Codes, and Formats (I 4.2)**
Map or translate local terminology, codes, and formats to standard terminology, codes, and formats to comply with health informatics standards. An EHR-S, which uses local terminology, must be capable of mapping and/or converting the local terminology into a standard terminology. For example, a local term or code for "ionized calcium" must be mapped to an equivalent, standardized (LOINC) term or code when archiving or exchanging artifacts.

Standards-Based Interoperability (I 5.0)

Provide automatic health delivery processes and seamless exchange of key clinical and administrative information through standards-based solutions. Interoperability standards enable an EHR-S to operate as a set of applications.

☐ **Interchange Standards (I 5.1)**
Support the ability to operate seamlessly with complementary systems by adherence to key interoperability standards. Systems may refer to other EHR-S, applications within an EHR-S, or other authorized entities that interact with an EHR-S. An EHR-S must adhere to standards for connectivity, information structures, and semantics—interoperability standards. An EHR-S, which may exist locally or remotely, must support seamless operations between complementary systems.

  ☐ An EHR-S must support realm-specific interoperability standards, such as:

    ☐ HL7 messages.

    ☐ Clinical document architecture (CDA).

☐   X12N healthcare transactions.

☐   Digital imaging and communication in medicine (DICOM).

☐   An EHR-S must be capable of common semantic representations to support information exchange.

☐   An EHR-S may use different standardized or local vocabularies in accordance with realm-specific requirements. In order to reconcile the semantic differences across vocabularies, an EHR-S must adhere to standard vocabulary or leverage vocabulary lookup and mapping capabilities that are included in the health informatics and terminology standards.

☐   An EHR-S must support multiple interaction modes to respond to differing levels of immediacy and types of exchange. For example, messaging is effective for many near real-time, asynchronous data exchange scenarios but may not be appropriate if the end user is requesting an immediate response from a remote application.

☐   An EHR-S may need to support the appropriate interaction mode in the case where store-and-forward, message-oriented interoperability is used. Examples include unsolicited event notification, query/response, query for display, unsolicited summary, and structured/discrete and unstructured clinical documents.

☐   **Standard-Based Application Integration (I 5.2)** .
Provide integration with complementary systems and infrastructure services, such as directory, vocabulary, etc, using standard based application programming interfaces, such as CCOW.[12] Similar to standard-based messaging, standard-based application integration requires that an EHR-S use standardized programming interfaces, where applicable. For example, CCOW may be used for visual integration and application of workflow management coalition (WfMC) standards for workflow integration.

☐   **Interchange Agreements (I 5.3)**
Support interaction with entity directories to determine the recipient's address profile and data exchange requirements and use these rules of interaction when exchanging information with partners. An EHR-S uses the entity registries to determine the security, addressing, and reliability requirements between partners. An EHR-S uses this information to define how data will be exchanged between the sender and the receiver.

Business Rules Management (I 6.0)

Manage the ability to create, update, delete, and version business rules, including institutional preferences. Apply business rules from necessary points within an EHR-S to control system behavior. An EHR-S audits changes made to business rules, as well as compliance to and overrides of applied business rules. An EHR-S business rule implementation functions include: decision support, diagnostic support, workflow control, access privileges, and system user defaults and preferences. An EHR-S supports the ability of providers and institutions to customize decision-support components, such as trigger, rules, or algorithms, as well as the wording of alerts and advice to meet realm-specific requirements and preferences. Examples of applied business rules include:

☐ Suggesting diagnosis based on the combination of symptoms, such as flu-like symptoms combined with widened mediastinum,[13] suggesting anthrax.

☐ Classifying a pregnant patient as a high risk due to factors such as age, health status, and prior pregnancy outcomes.

☐ Sending an update to an immunization registry when a vaccination is administered.

☐ Limiting access to mental health information to a patient's psychiatrist/ psychologist.

☐ Establishing system level defaults, such as for vocabulary data sets to be implemented.

☐ Establishing user level preferences, such as allowing the use of health information for research purposes.

Workflow Management (I 7.0)

Support workflow management functions, including both the management and setup of work queues, personnel, and system interfaces, as well as the implementation functions that use workflow-related business rules to direct the flow of work assignments. Workflow management functions that an EHR-S supports include:

☐ Distribution of information to and from internal and external parties.

☐ Support for task management and parallel and serial task distribution.

☐ Support for notification and task routing based on system triggers.

☐ Support for task assignments, escalations, and redirection in accordance with business rules.

Workflow definitions and management may be implemented by a designated application or distributed across an EHR-S.

SUMMARY

The EHR-DSTU is subject to testing into the summer of 2006, at which time HL7 will vote to convert from DSTU to approved standard status. From July 2004 until the close of the testing period, physicians have an opportunity to test EHR components that are described in this chapter and to make comments to HL7 concerning specifics and relevancy to the conduct of business in their practices. Directions for providing comments appear at the beginning of this chapter in the section, "Directions for Physician Input." We urge you to send your comments to HL7, as such comments will enhance the content and value to your business of the approved EHR functional descriptors.

We also urge you to follow developments pertaining to EHRs in the media, as they are evolving rapidly, driven by a combination of federal government interest in EHRs and increasing vendor interest in providing innovative digital clinical and administrative tools comprising EHR components to physicians. "Although President Bush has called for widespread EHR adoption within 10 years, Brailer said he told Bush that the goal could be accomplished within seven years. He said the main challenge would involve getting EHR adoption to the 'tipping point,' when about 45% to 50% of the market is using the records, rather than 100% of the market."[14]

There is increasing evidence that EHR systems are catching on and that more rapid adoption may occur in the market. For example, a recent article indicates that "nearly four in 10 physicians have an EHR system in place or are implementing one, according to a recent member survey by the American Academy of Family Physicians (AAFP). Of the respondents who have EHRs in place, 73% said such systems helped to improve patient health by reducing prescribing errors and enhancing patient communication. In addition, 65% of physicians with an EHR used decision support tools like up-to-the-minute research and treatment guidelines to reference patient health information. About half of all respondents said they wanted to purchase an EHR, with 15% planning to implement the system within one year and 16% within two years."[15]

There also is increasing evidence that EMR and EHR systems are challenging to implement, but delivering returns on investment (ROI). With regard to the challenge, one study suggests that success is based on implementing the following steps[16]:

- Assess change readiness
- Map out the workflow
- Set realistic expectations
- Get physicians involved
- Avoid training shortcuts
- Show early wins
- Keep an eye on the prize

In the first part of this book, we provided a variety of tools for you to use for meeting the challenge.

With regard to ROI, this study goes on to say that potential benefits of EMR and EHR systems "include streamlined workflow, elimination of costly chart pulls and transcription, regained revenue via correct coding, faster insurance reimbursement and more—and its potential return can wind up being three to four times what the practice paid to invest in it."[16] Two other studies also illustrate the growing number of stories about achieving returns on investment:

- "Mark Neaman, president and CEO of Evanston Northwestern Healthcare (ENH) . . . said that successful EHR implementation is a monumental task that requires enterprisewide commitment. ENH recently launched a $30 million EHR system and has seen 'impressive' benefits. The turnaround time in obtaining test results has fallen significantly, and entire categories of medication errors and potential errors have been eliminated, Neaman said. In addition, delayed administration of patient medication has decreased by 70%, and omitted administration of medication has dropped 20%."[17]

- Colorado Otolaryngology's electronic records system—from Oak Ridge, Tennessee-based All Meds—provided a return on investment in many different ways. The practice was able to reduce administrative staff then increase staffing in revenue-producing areas such as nursing, triage and out-of-office scheduling. 'There is no doubt that electronic records improve patient care, and if you look at it purely from a business perspective, there's no way you can run a viable business any more without having them,' [J. Lewis] Romett [president of the Colorado Springs-based practice] said."[18]

In addition to the returns on investment, there are motivational factors that are now and will in the future make digital processes in the practice a reality. A recent survey reported the following:

- The top three factors motivating healthcare organizations to implement an electronic health record (EHR) are the need to: improve clinical processes or workflow efficiency, improve quality of care, and share patient-record information among practitioners, according to a survey by the Medical Records Institute, Boston. The responses, gathered early this summer from 436 providers, also indicate the biggest barriers: lack of funding, inability to find an affordable EHR, and lack of medical staff support.[19]

With regard to the barriers encountered, we have seen in this book that the federal government is focused on exploring initiatives for providing financial incentives for adoption of EMR and EHR systems, and for making EMR and EHR systems more affordable, such as licensing SNOMED-CT for use by the US healthcare industry at no cost. With regard to "lack of medical staff support," we hope that the tools that we have provided in this book, along with workforce *champions* in your practice, will help to make adoption and implementation of EMR and EHR systems in your practice a reality with a positive ROI.

Finally, we urge you to keep up with developments in this fast paced world of digital processes in healthcare. Visiting any of the Web sites that we have identified in the book, and especially with the citations in this chapter, will keep you informed. In addition to the resources at the American Medical Association (AMA), we also commend to your attention the resources of the American Health Information Management Association's *Journal of AHIMA* (www.ahima.org), *Modern Healthcare* (www.modernhealthcare.com), and the California Healthcare Foundation's *iHealth Beat* (www.ihealthbeat.org).

Let us know how you are doing.

ENDNOTES

1. Thompson launches "decade of health information technology" [news release]. Washington, DC: US Department of Health and Human Services; July 21, 2004. Available at: www.hhs.gov/news/press/2004pres/20040721a.html.

2. HIT report at-a-glance [fact sheet]. Washington, DC: US Department of Health and Human Services; July 21, 2004. Available at: www.hhs.gov/news/press/2004pres/20040721.html.

3. Secretary Thompson, seeking fastest possible results, names first health information technology coordinator [news release]. Washington, DC: US Department of Health and Human Services; May 6, 2004. Available at: www.hhs.gov/news/press/2004pres/20040506.html.

4. Heffler S, et al. Health Spending Projections Through 2013. *Health Affairs-Web Exclusive*. February 11, 2004:W4-80. Available at: www.healthaffairs.org.

5. "Established in 1987, Health Level Seven (HL7) is an [American National Standards Institute] ANSI accredited, not-for-profit standard-development organization, whose mission is to provide standards for the exchange, integration, sharing, and retrieval of electronic health information; support clinical practice; and support the management, delivery, and evaluation of health services. ANSI accreditation, coupled with HL7's own procedures, dictates that any standard published by HL7 and submitted to ANSI for approval, be developed and ratified by a process that adheres to ANSI's procedures for open consensus and meets a balance of interest requirement by attaining near equal participation in the voting process by the various constituencies that are materially affected by the standard. . . ." See Dickinson G, Fischetti L, Heard S. *HL7 EHR System Functional Model: Draft Standard for Trial Use.* Ann Arbor, Mich: Health Level Seven, Inc; 2004.

6. For more information go to: www.hl7.org and refer to "HL7 EHR System Functional Model: Draft Standard for Trial Use" and "HL7 Board of Directors Unanimously Approves EHR for Draft Standard Status" under *Recent News.*

7. The foundation for this function is a technical specification (TS) of the International Organization for Standardization (ISO), titled *ISO/TS 18308:2004: Health Informatics—Requirements for an Electronic Health Record Architecture* (January 22, 2004, 28 pages). "The purpose of ISO/TS 18308:2004 is to assemble and collate a set of clinical and technical requirements for an

electronic health record architecture (EHRA) that supports using, sharing, and exchanging electronic health records across different health sectors, different countries, and different models of healthcare delivery. It gives requirements for the architecture but not the specifications of the architecture itself." For more information on ISO/TS 18308: 2004, go to: www.iso.org/iso/en/CatalogueDetailPage.CatalogueDetail?CSNUMBER=33397&ICS1=35&ICS2=240&ICS3=80.

8. The Administrative Simplification privacy and security standards required under the Health Insurance Portability and Accountability Act (HIPAA) are outlined in *HIPAA Plain & Simple: A Compliance Guide for Healthcare Professionals* by Carolyn P. Hartley and Edward D. Jones (AMA Press, 2003).

9. This supports the function, Manage Consents and Authorizations (DC 1.5.1).

10. For a description of these terminologies, see Chapter 5.

11. X12 is an accredited standards committee (ASC) organization under auspices of the American National Standards Institute (ANSI) that has been responsible for defining the implementation specifications for the HIPAA Administrative Simplification transaction and code set standards.

12. CCOW (clinical context object workgroup) is a vendor-independent standard developed by the HL7 organization to allow clinical applications to share information at the point of care. For more information go to: www.ccow-info.com.

13. "The space in the chest between the pleural sacs of the lungs that contains all the tissues and organs of the chest except the lungs and pleurae." *Merriam-Webster's Collegiate Dictionary*. 11th ed. Springfield, Mass: Merriam-Webster, Inc; 2003:770.

14. Government's health IT goals should be accomplished in seven years. *Health-IT World News*. August 5, 2004. Available at: www.ihealthbeat.org.

15. Physician practices: EHRs gain ground with doctors. *Health Management Technology*. September, 2004:10. Available at: www.healthmgttech.com.

16. Koo CC. Getting ready for an EMR: physician practices should consider several key factors before selecting an electronic medical record system. *Health Management Technology*. August, 2004:26–28. Available at: www.healthmgttech.com.

17. Electronic health records: expert—look closely to find the ROI in EHRs. *Health Management Technology*. August, 2004:8. Available at: www.healthmgttech.com.

18. Doc: electronic records not a choice. *Health Data Technology*. November, 2004:26. Available at: www.healthdatamanagement.com.

19. Van Beusekom M. EHR: why or why not? *Healthcare Informatics*. October, 2004:80. Available at: www.healthcare-informatics.com. (The survey on which the results are based is available at: www.medrecinst.com.)

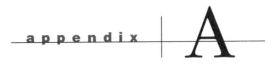
US Department of Health and Human Services News Release: HHS Launches New Efforts to Promote Paperless Health Care System

Tuesday, July 1, 2003

HHS Launches New Efforts to Promote Paperless Health Care System[1]

Department of Health and Human Services (HHS) Secretary Tommy G. Thompson today announced two new steps in building a national electronic healthcare system that will allow patients and their doctors to access their complete medical records anytime and anywhere they are needed, leading to reduced medical errors, improved patient care, and reduced healthcare costs.

First, the Secretary announced that the Department has signed an agreement with the College of American Pathologists (CAP) to license the College's standardized medical vocabulary system and make it available without charge throughout the US. This action opens the door to establishing a common medical language as a key element in building a unified electronic medical records system in the US.

Secondly, the Secretary announced that HHS has commissioned the Institute of Medicine to design a standardized model of an electronic health record. The healthcare standards development organization known as Health Level Seven (HL7) has been asked to evaluate the model once it has been designed. HHS will share the standardized model record at no cost with all components of the US healthcare system. The Department expects to have a model record ready in 2004.

Today's announcements are part of the ongoing HHS effort to develop the National Health Information Infrastructure by encouraging and facilitating the widespread use of modern information technology to improve the nation's healthcare system.

"Banks and other financial institutions all across the country can talk to each other electronically, which has streamlined customer transactions and reduced errors," Secretary Thompson said. "We want to do the same thing for the American healthcare system. We want to build a standardized platform on which physicians' offices, insurance companies, hospitals and others can all communicate electronically, which will improve patient care while reducing the medical errors and the high costs plaguing our healthcare system."

With terms for more than 340,000 medical concepts, the College's standardized system has been recognized as the world's most comprehensive clinical terminology database available. The licensing agreement with the CAP will make it possible for healthcare providers, hospitals, insurance companies, public health departments, medical research facilities, and others to easily incorporate this uniform terminology system into their information systems.

"This system will prove invaluable in facilitating the automated exchange of clinical information needed to protect patient safety, detect emerging public health threats, better coordinate patient care, and compile research data for patients participating in clinical trials," Secretary Thompson said.

The CAP agreement announced today will be administered through the National Library of Medicine (NLM), a component of HHS' National Institutes of Health (NIH). NLM has issued a five-year, $32.4 million contract to the College for a permanent license for their terminology, known as SNOMED (Systematized Nomenclature of Medicine) Clinical Terms. The licensing agreement includes the core database in both English and Spanish along with regular updates. The terms of the contract include a one-time payment—shared by the Department of Veterans Affairs, the Department of Defense, and many HHS agencies—with annual update fees to be borne by the NLM.

"Today we take a bold step by making SNOMED available, a critical step in adopting health information standards across the federal government," Secretary of Veterans Affairs Anthony J. Principi said. "Putting health information standards in the public domain and promptly adopting health information standards for the federal health partners, is the 'tipping point' for national standards that strengthen our electronic health record systems, help optimize our healthcare, and, most importantly, improve the health of veterans as well as all of the people of the US."

"The Department of Defense is pleased to have contributed to the government-wide effort to license SNOMED. This effort will enable us to better share health information within the Federal government and beyond. I am delighted with our Federal partnership in this important step toward improving healthcare for all Americans," said Dr Winkenwerder, assistant secretary of defense for health affairs.

"This license validates the College's longstanding support for the development of medical standards like SNOMED to further improve the quality of healthcare. It ensures that government and the private sector entities in the US will be able to use a common approach to clinical coding, making it easier to coordinate care and exchange needed information," said Paul A. Raslavicus, MD, president of the CAP.

The contract between NLM and the College of American Pathologists comes after three years of negotiations. The effort was supported by all the agencies participating in the Consolidated Health Informatics initiative (CHI), which is working to adopt government-wide standards for clinical health data. CHI is the healthcare component of President Bush's eGov Initiatives, created under the President's Management Agenda, to make it easier for citizens and businesses to interact with the government, save taxpayer dollars and streamline citizen-to-government transactions. More information on CHI and the President's eGov Initiatives may be found at www.egov.gov.

NLM will distribute SNOMED through its Unified Medical Language System, which incorporates, links, and distributes in a common format 100 different biomedical and health vocabularies and classifications. Details of the SNOMED license arrangement as well as information on obtaining access to the SNOMED database may be found at: www.nlm. nih.gov/research/umls/Snomed/snomed_announcement.html.

ENDNOTE

1. This news release can be accessed at: www.hhs.gov/news/press/ 2003pres/20030701.html.

Health IT Strategic Framework: Executive Summary

On April 27, 2004, President Bush called for widespread adoption of interoperable electronic health records (EHRs) within 10 years, and also established the position of National Coordinator for Health Information Technology. On May 6, 2004, Secretary Tommy G. Thompson appointed David J. Brailer, MD, PhD, to serve in this new position. The federal government has already played an active role in the evolution and use of health information technology (HIT), including adoption and ongoing support for standards needed to achieve interoperability. Executive Order 13335 requires the National Coordinator to report within 90 days of operation on the development and implementation of a strategic plan to guide the nationwide implementation of HIT in both the public and private sectors.

In fulfilling the requirements of the Executive Order, this report outlines a framework for a strategic plan that will be dynamic, iterative, and implemented in coordination with the private sector.[1] In addition, this report includes attachments from the Office of Personnel Management (OPM), the Department of Defense (DoD), and the Department of Veterans Affairs (VA). Collectively, this report and related attachments represent the progress to date on the development and implementation of a comprehensive HIT strategic plan.

READINESS FOR CHANGE

There is a great need for information tools to be used in the delivery of health care. Preventable medical errors and treatment variations have recently gained attention. Clinicians may not know the latest treatment options, and practices vary across clinicians and regions. Consumers want to ensure that they have choices in treatment, and when they do, they want to have the information they need to make decisions about their care. Concerns about the privacy and security of personal medical information remain high. Public health monitoring, bioterror surveillance, research, and quality monitoring require data that depends on the widespread adoption of HIT.

VISION FOR CONSUMER-CENTRIC AND INFORMATION-RICH CARE

Many envision a health care industry that is consumer centric and information-rich, in which medical information follows the consumer, and information tools guide medical decisions. Clinicians have appropriate access to a patient's complete treatment history, including medical records, medication history, laboratory results, and radiographs, among other information. Clinicians order medications with computerized systems that eliminate handwriting errors and automatically check for doses that are too high or too low, for harmful interactions with other drugs, and for allergies. Prescriptions are also checked against the health plan's formulary, and the out-of-pocket costs of the prescribed drug can be compared with alternative treatments. Clinicians receive electronic reminders in the form of alerts about treatment procedures and medical guidelines. This is a different way of delivering health care than that which currently exists, but one that many have envisioned. This new way will result in fewer medical errors, fewer unnecessary treatments or wasteful care, and fewer variations in care, and will ultimately improve care for all Americans. Care will be centered around the consumer and will be delivered electronically as well as in person. Clinicians can spend more time on patient care, and employers will gain productivity and competitive benefits from health care spending.

Strategic Framework

In order to realize a new vision for health care made possible through the use of information technology, strategic actions embraced by the public and private health sectors need to be taken over many years. There are four major goals that will be pursued in realizing this vision for improved health care. Each of these goals has a corresponding set of strategies and related specific actions that will advance and focus future efforts. These goals and strategies are summarized below.

Goal 1: Inform Clinical Practice

Informing clinical practice is fundamental to improving care and making health care delivery more efficient. This goal centers largely around efforts to bring EHRs directly into clinical practice. This will reduce medical errors and duplicative work, and enable clinicians to focus their efforts more directly on improved patient care. Three strategies for realizing this goal are:

■ *Strategy 1. Incentivize EHR adoption.* The transition to safe, more consumer-friendly and regionally integrated care delivery will re-quire shared investments in information tools and changes to current clinical practice.

■ *Strategy 2. Reduce risk of EHR investment.* Clinicians who purchase EHRs and who attempt to change their clinical practices and office operations face a variety of risks that make this decision unduly challenging. Low-cost support systems that reduce risk, failure, and partial use of EHRs are needed.

■ *Strategy 3. Promote EHR diffusion in rural and underserved areas.* Practices and hospitals in rural and other underserved areas lag in EHR adoption. Technology transfer and other support efforts are needed to ensure widespread adoption.

Goal 2: Interconnect Clinicians

Interconnecting clinicians will allow information to be portable and to move with consumers from one point of care to another. This will require an interoperable infrastructure to help clinicians get access to critical health care information when their clinical and/or treatment decisions are being made. The three strategies for realizing this goal are:

■ *Strategy 1. Foster regional collaborations.* Local oversight of health information exchange that reflects the needs and goals of a population should be developed.

■ *Strategy 2. Develop a national health information network.* A set of common intercommunication tools such as mobile authen-tication, Web services architecture, and security technologies are needed to support data movement that is inexpensive and secure. A national health information network that can provide low-cost and secure data movement is needed, along with a public-private oversight or management function to ensure adherence to public policy objectives.

■ *Strategy 3. Coordinate federal health information systems.* There is a need for federal health information systems to be interoperable and to exchange data so that federal care delivery, reimbursement, and oversight are more efficient and cost-effective. Federal health in-formation systems will be interoperable and consistent with the national health information network.

Goal 3: Personalize Care

Consumer-centric information helps individuals manage their own wellness and assists with their personal health care decisions. The ability to personalize care is a critical component of using health care information in a meaningful manner. The three strategies for realizing this goal are:

- *Strategy 1. Encourage use of Personal Health Records.* Consumers are increasingly seeking information about their care as a means of getting better control over their health care experience, and PHRs that provide customized facts and guidance to them are needed.

- *Strategy 2. Enhance informed consumer choice.* Consumers should have the ability to select clinicians and institutions based on what they value and the information to guide their choice, including but not limited to, the quality of care providers deliver.

- *Strategy 3. Promote use of telehealth systems.* The use of telehealth—remote communication technologies—can provide access to health services for consumers and clinicians in rural and underserved areas. Telehealth systems that can support the delivery of health care services when the participants are in different locations are needed.

Goal 4: Improve Population Health

Population health improvement requires the collection of timely, accurate, and detailed clinical information to allow for the evaluation of health care delivery and the reporting of critical findings to public health officials, clinical trials and other research, and feedback to clinicians. Three strategies for realizing this goal are:

- *Strategy 1. Unify public health surveillance architectures.* An interoperable public health surveillance system is needed that will allow exchange of information, consistent with current law, between provider organizations, organizations they contract with, and state and federal agencies.

- *Strategy 2. Streamline quality and health status monitoring.* Many different state and local organizations collect subsets of data for specific purposes and use it in different ways. A streamlined quality-monitoring infrastructure that will allow for a complete look at quality and other issues in real-time and at the point of care is needed.

- *Strategy 3. Accelerate research and dissemination of evidence.* Information tools are needed that can accelerate scientific discoveries and their translation into clinically useful products, applications, and knowledge.

KEY ACTIONS

The Framework for Strategic Action will guide the development of a full strategic plan for widespread HIT adoption. At the same time, a variety of key actions that have begun to implement this strategy are underway, including:

- *Establishing a Health Information Technology Leadership Panel to evaluate the urgency of investments and recommend immediate actions.* As many different options and policies are considered for financing HIT adoption, the Secretary of HHS is taking immediate action by forming a Health Information Technology Leadership Panel, consisting of executives and leaders. This panel will assess the costs and benefits of HIT to industry and society, and evaluate the urgency of investments in these tools. These leaders will discuss the immediate steps for both the public and private sector to take with regard to HIT adoption, based on their individual business experience. The Health Information Technology Leadership Panel will deliver a synthesized report comprised of these options to the Secretary no later than Fall 2004.

- *Private sector certification of health information technology products.* EHRs and even specific components such as decision support software are unique among clinical tools in that they do not need to meet minimal standards to be used to deliver care. To increase uptake of EHRs and reduce the risk of product implementation failure, the federal government is exploring ways to work with the private sector to develop minimal product standards for EHR functionality, interoperability, and security. A private sector ambulatory EHR certification task force is determining the feasibility of certification of EHR products based on functionality, security, and interoperability.

- *Funding community health information exchange demonstrations.* A health information exchange program through Health Resources and Services Administration, Office of the Advancement of Telehealth (HRSA/OAT) has a cooperative agreement with the Foundation for eHealth Initiative to administer contracts to support the Connecting Communities for Better Health (CCBH) Program totaling $2.3 million. This program is providing seed funds and support to multi-stakeholder collaboratives within communities (both geographic and non-geographic) to implement health information exchanges, including the formation of regional health information organizations (RHIOs) to drive improvements in health care quality, safety, and efficiency. The specific communities that will receive the funding through this program will be announced and recognized during the Secretarial Summit on July 21.

- *Planning the formation of a private interoperability consortium.* To begin the process of movement toward a national health information network, HHS is releasing a request for information (RFI) in the summer of 2004 inviting responses describing the requirements for private sector consortia that would form to plan, develop, and operate a health information network. Members of the consortium would agree to participate in the governance structure and activities and finance the consortium in an equitable manner. The role that HHS could play in facilitating the work of the consortium and assisting in identifying the services that the consortium would provide will be explored, including the standards to which the health information network would adhere to in order to ensure that public policy goals are executed and that rapid adoption of interoperable EHRs is advanced. The Federal Health Architecture (FHA) will be coordinated and interoperable with the national health information network.

- *Requiring standards to facilitate electronic prescribing.* CMS will be proposing a regulation that will require the first set of widely adopted e-prescribing standards in preparation for the implementation of the new Medicare drug benefit in 2006. When this regulation is final, Medicare Prescription Drug Plan (PDP) Sponsors will be required to offer e-prescribing, which will significantly drive adoption across the United States. Health plans and pharmacy benefit managers that are PDP sponsors could work with RHIOs, including physician offices, to implement private industry-certified interoperable e-prescribing tools and to train and support clinicians.

- *Establishing a Medicare beneficiary portal.* An immediate step in improving consumer access to personal and customized health information is CMS' Medicare Beneficiary Portal, which provides secure health information via the Internet. This portal will be hosted by a private company under contract with CMS, and will enable authorized Medicare beneficiaries to have access to their information online or by calling 1-800-MEDICARE. Initially the portal will provide access to fee-for-service claims information, which includes claims type, dates of service, and procedures. The pilot test for the portal will be conducted for the residents of Indiana. In the near term, CMS plans to expand the portal to include prevention information in the form of reminders to beneficiaries to schedule their Medicare-covered preventive health care services. CMS also plans to work toward providing additional electronic health information tools to beneficiaries for their use in improving their health.

- *Sharing clinical research data through a secure infrastructure.* FDA and NIH, together with the Clinical Data Interchange Standards Consortium (CDISC), a consortium of over 40 pharmaceutical companies and clinical research organizations, have developed a standard for representing observations made in clinical trials called the Study Data Tabulation Model (SDTM). This model will facilitate the automation of the largely paper-based clinical research process, which will lead to greater efficiencies in industry and government-sponsored clinical research. The first release of the model and associated implementation guide will be finalized prior to the July 21 Secretarial Summit and represents an important step by government, academia, and industry in working together to accelerate research through the use of standards and HIT.

- *Commitment to standards.* A key component of progress in interoperable health information is the development of technically sound and robustly specified interoperability standards and policies. There have been considerable efforts by HHS, DoD, and VA to adopt health information standards for use by all federal health agencies. As part of the Consolidated Health Informatics (CHI) initiative, the agencies have agreed to endorse 20 sets of standards to make it easier for information to be shared across agencies and to serve as a model for the private sector. Additionally, the Public Health Information Network (PHIN) and the National Electronic Disease Surveillance System (NEDSS), under the leadership of the Centers for Disease Control and Prevention (CDC), have made notable progress in development of shared data models, data standards, and controlled vocabularies for electronic laboratory reporting and health information exchange. With HHS support, Health Level 7 (HL7) has also created a functional model and standards for the EHR.

PUBLIC-PRIVATE PARTNERSHIP

Leaders across the public and private sector recognize that the adoption and effective use of HIT requires a joint effort between federal, state, and local governments and the private sector. The value of HIT will be best realized under the conditions of a competitive technology industry, privately operated support services, choice among clinicians and provider organizations, and payers who reward clinicians based on quality. The Federal government has already played an active role in the evolution and use of HIT. In FY04, total federal spending on HIT was more than $900 million. Initiatives range from supporting research in advanced HIT to the development and use of EHR systems. Much of this work demonstrates that HIT can be used effectively in supporting health care delivery and improving quality and patient safety.

ROLE OF THE NATIONAL COORDINATOR FOR HEALTH INFORMATION TECHNOLOGY

Executive Order 13335 directed the appointment of the National Coordinator for Health Information Technology to coordinate programs and policies regarding HIT across the federal government. The National Coordinator was charged with directing HIT programs within HHS and coordinating them with those of other relevant Executive Branch agencies. In fulfillment of this, the National Coordinator has taken responsibility for the National Health Information Infrastructure Initiative (NHII), the FHA, and the Consolidated Health Informatics Initiative (CHI), and is currently assessing other health information technology programs and efforts. In addition, the National Coordinator was charged with coordinating outreach and consultation between the federal government and the private sector. As part of this, the National Coordinator was directed to coordinate with the National Committee on Vital Health Statistics (NCVHS) and other advisory committees.

The National Coordinator will collaborate with DoD, VA, and OPM to encourage the widespread adoption of HIT throughout the health care system. To do this, the National Coordinator will gather and disseminate the lessons learned from both DoD and VA in successfully incorporating HIT into the delivery of health care, and facilitate the development and transfer of knowledge and technology to the private sector. OPM, as the purchaser of health care for the federal government, has a unique role and the ability to encourage the use of EHRs through the Federal Employees Health Benefits Program, and the National Coordinator will assist in gaining the complementary alignment of OPM policies with those of the private sector.

REPORTS FROM OPM, DOD, AND VA

The Executive Order also directs the OPM, the DoD, and the VA to submit reports on HIT to the President through the Secretary of Health and Human Services. These reports are included in this report as Attachments 1 through 3.

OPM administers the Federal Employees Health Benefits Program for the federal government and the more than eight million people it covers. As the nation's largest purchaser of health benefits, OPM is keenly interested in high-quality care and reasonable cost. The adoption of an interoperable HIT infrastructure is a key to achieving both. OPM is currently exploring a variety of options to leverage its purchasing power and alliances to move the adoption of HIT forward. OPM will be strongly encouraging health plans to promote the early adoption of HIT. Details on these options can be found in OPM's report, "Federal Employees Health Benefits Program Initiatives to Promote the Use of Health Information Technology" (Attachment 1).[2]

The VA, collaboratively with DoD, provides joint recommendations to address the special needs of these populations (Attachment 2).[3] As mirrored in the DoD Report (Attachment 3),[4] these recommendations focus on the capture of lessons learned, the knowledge and technology transfers to be gained from successful VA/DoD data exchange initiatives, the adoption of common standards and terminologies to promote more effective and rapid development of health technologies, and the development of telehealth technologies to improve care in rural and remote areas.

The DoD has significant experience in delivering care in isolated conditions such as those encountered in wartime or overseas peacekeeping missions, which can be compared to the conditions in some rural health care environments. Examples of the technologies used in these conditions include telehealth for radiology, mental health, dermatology, pathology, and dental consultations; online personalized health records for beneficiary use; bed regulation for disaster planning; basic patient encounter documentation; pharmacy, radiology, and laboratory order entry and results retrieval for use in remote areas and small clinics; pharmacy, radiology, and laboratory order entry and results retrieval; admissions and discharges; appointments for use in small hospitals; and online education offerings for health care providers. Technology products, outcomes, benefits, and cumulative knowledge will be shared for use within the private sector and local/state organizations to help guide their planning efforts (see Attachment 3 for more details).

The VA's report, "Approaches to Make Health Information Systems Available and Affordable to Rural and Medically Underserved Communities" (Attachment 2), also highlights its successful strategy to develop high-quality EHR technologies that remain in the public domain. These technologies may be suitable for transfer to rural and medically underserved settings. VA's primary health information systems and EHR (VistA and the Computerized Patient Record System [the current system] and HealtheVet-VistA, the next generation in development) provide leading government/public-owned health information technologies that support the provision, measurement, and improvement of quality, affordable care across 1300 VA inpatient and ambulatory settings. The VA continues to make a version of VistA available in the public domain as a means of fostering widespread development of high-performance EHR systems. The VA is also incorporating the CHI approved standards into its next-generation HealtheVet-VistA. Furthermore, the VA is developing PHR technologies such as My HealtheVet, which are consistent with the larger strategic goal of making veterans (persons) the center of health care. Finally, the VA's health information technologies, such as bar code medication administration, VistA Imaging, and telehealth applications, provide the VA with exceptional tools that improve patient safety and enable the increasingly geographically dispersed provision of care to patients in all settings. These and other technologies are proposed as federal technology transfer options in furtherance of the President's goals.

CONCLUSION

Health information technology has the potential to transform health care delivery, bringing information where it is needed and refocusing health care around the consumer. This can be done without substantial regulation or industry upheaval. It can give us both better care—care that is higher in quality, safer, and more consumer responsive—and more efficient care—care that is less wasteful, more appropriate, and more available. The changes that will accompany the full use of information technology in the health care industry will pose challenges to longstanding assumptions and practices. However, these changes are needed, beneficial, and inevitable. Action should be taken now to achieve the benefits of HIT. A well-planned and coordinated effort, sustained over a number of years, can deliver results that will better support America's health care professionals and better serve the public.

ENDNOTES

1. The full Health IT Strategic Framework can be accessed at: www.hhs.gov/healthit/frameworkchapters.html. The Executive Summary can be accessed at: www.hhs.gov/healthit/executivesummary.html.

2. Attachment 1 can be accessed at: www.hhs.gov/healthit/attachment_1.

3. Attachment 2 can be accessed at: www.hhs.gov/healthit/attachment_2/attachment_2.html.

4. Attachment 3 can be accessed at: www.hhs.gov/healthit/attachment_3/attachment_3.html.

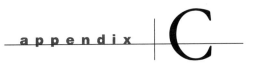

Information Technology Trends and Solutions: 2004 Summary Report

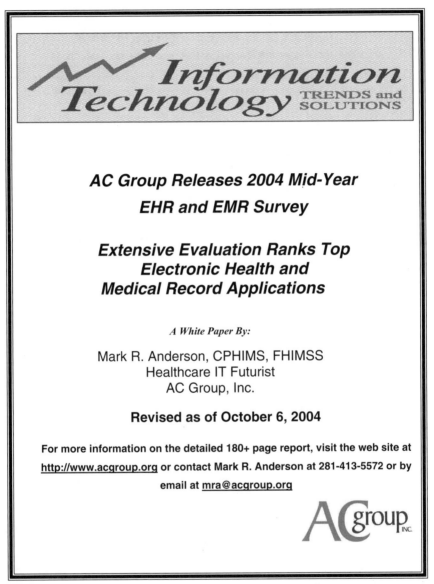

AC GROUP RELEASES 2004 MID YEAR EMR/EHR SURVEY
Extensive Evaluation Ranks Top EHR and EMR Applications

San Francisco, CA (October 2, 2004) – AC Group, Inc. (ACG) released their fourth report on **Electronic Medical Record (EMR)** and **Electronic Health Record (EHR)** applications today at the MGMA conference in San Francisco. This year's mid-year report provides physicians with one of the most comprehensive evaluations to date of leading EMR/EHR applications. According to the author, Mark Anderson, Healthcare IT Futurist, "Physicians are looking for a 3rd party independent evaluation of the various EMR/EHR offerings in the marketplace today. The current pressures in the industry for increased efficiency and better care delivery, coupled with significant advances in technology and applications, have enabled EMRs to take center stage. The challenge with EMRs is that it is very difficult for the average physician practice to effectively evaluate its' options." The survey is an extensive evaluation of functional criteria that can serve as a valuable tool for the vendor selection process. The entire report is over 180 pages long and covers all 6 levels of technology for the physician's office.

Summary Results: To insure that the application met the real needs of physicians, a detailed study was conducted by AC Group, Inc. during the Spring of 2002, 2003, 2004 and then again in October of 2003 and 2004. The AC Group EMR report is based on 34 months of research and the cumulative results of their 90-page questionnaire that included 5,455 functional questions divided into 27 categories and 4 methods of operations. The four methods of operation included:

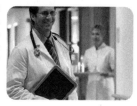

1. Desktop capability (1,718 questions)
2. Wireless capability (1,447 questions)
3. Remote access capability (1,418 questions)
4. PDA and mobile capability (872 questions)

The 27 functional categories included sections on the Institute of Medicine's (IOM) requirements for a computerized patient record (CPR), along with functional questions relating to operational areas including prescriptions, charge capture, dictation, interface with laboratories, physician order entry, decision support and alerts, security, personal health records, reporting and documentation. The EMR/EHR evaluation included a weighted point value for each of the 5,455 question based on the following criteria:

○   The current product **doesn't** offer this functionality
○   The current product **provides** the functionality for an **additional cost**
○   The current product **provides** the functionality from **a third party**
○   A future product enhancement in the **next three months** will provide the functionality
○   A future product enhancement in the **next six months** will provide the functionality
○   A future product enhancement in the **next year** will provide the functionality
○   The product **provides** the functionality currently

AC GROUP RELEASES 2004 MID YEAR EMR/EHR SURVEY
Extensive Evaluation Ranks Top EHR and EMR Applications

For the first time, the 2004 report includes a point system based on a combination of functionality, company size, client base, end-user satisfaction, and price. This will provide a more comprehensive view of the ability of the end user to derive benefits from the product. Through our research, we have learned that while having the appropriate level of functionality is critical, providers require a vendor that will support and continue to develop the product. Each area was given a weighted value, and each vendor was assigned a "Total Weighted Point Value". Additionally in the October 2004 report, AC Group divided the rankings based on the type of product:

O **Certified EHR** – Rating of over 85%. Full EMR with national drug and clinical alerts, national clinical protocols and guidelines, 3rd party clinical knowledge base, clinical decision support, clinical standards, physician specific summary page with workflow. Includes multi-Healthplan specific health maintenance rules, medical necessarily checking, formulary compliance. An EHR also includes patient direct interaction with their own Personal Health Record (PHR) via the internet or in-office kiosks. Certified EHR vendors already meet al of the requirements of certified EMR and Charting systems.

O **Certified EMR** - Rating of over 70%. Full Charting system with automated E & M coding, drug alerts, limited national knowledgebase and clinical decision support, limited formulary compliance, summary of patient specific clinical results on one page.

O **Charting System** – Complete clinical notes with limited alerts and limited clinical decision support. Limited E & M coding methodology, limited summary of patient clinical results on summary page.

O **EMR Lite Application** – Limited clinical note, e-prescribing, limited document image management, clinical results tracking and messaging, viewing of lab results and dictated reports.

Overall, four companies, **NextGen, Epic, Allscripts, and Cerner** received the highest overall total rating. Three important caveats to keep in mind as you review the results:

1. Literally hundreds of products are identified as EMRs, and while a good faith effort was made to contact as many vendors as possible, many chose not to respond.

2. The survey findings are based on what *vendors* said about their *own* products.

3. Fourteen of the time vendors were required to participate in face-to-face demonstrations of their product's functionality in order to receive "certification". The certification process tested more than 200 scenarios.

4. A few of the highly visible EMR vendors elected NOT to participate in the survey. Many of these vendors are not willing to document their functionality in writing, while others state that either they do not participate in surveys or they were too busy to participate.

When evaluating functionality by different methods of input, the ACG team determined that today's technology allows end-users the same functionality no matter where they are located. In 95% of the cases, the vendor's application functioned the same on the desktop, from a remote location, and from a wireless tablet. Therefore, the EMR evaluation

AC GROUP RELEASES 2004 MID YEAR EMR/EHR SURVEY
Extensive Evaluation Ranks Top EHR and EMR Applications

team was able to consolidate Desktop, Remote and Wireless functionality into one rating. The only major difference was the functionality on a PDA device – given that the screen size is limited. Therefore the EMR team created a separate rating for PDA devices. Simply stated, a number of the vendors that were highly ranked for the triad of desktop, remote and wireless, either did not offer a portable device or had one with limited functionality. When their overall performance ranking included low or nil scores for PDA their ranking dropped precipitously. The vendors that participated in this year's evaluation or had participated in one of our prior evaluations included:

- A4 Health Systems
- AllMeds
- Allscripts Healthcare Solutions
- Alteer
- Amazing Charts
- Amicore
- Axolotl
- Bizmatics
- Bond Technologies
- Cerner
- Chartcare, Inc.
- Chartlogic
- Cliniflow (Monarch)
- Dr Notes
- eClinicalworks
- e-MDS
- EPIC

- GE Medical Systems Information Tech.
- Greenway Medical Technologies
- Hamilton Assoc
- Healthvision
- InteGreat, Inc.
- iMedica Corp.
- JMJ Technologies
- McKesson
- MDAnywhere
- MEDCOM Information Systems, Inc.
- Medical Information Systems, Inc.
- Medical Office Online
- MedInformatix
- Medinotes
- MediNotes Corporation
- MedNet System
- MeridianEMR

- Misys Healthcare Systems
- NextGen Healthcare Information Systems
- Noteworthy Medical Systems
- OmniMD
- Orion Systems International Inc
- Physician Micro Systems, Inc.
- PraxisEMR (infor-Med)
- Smart Doctor
- SynaMed
- Task Technologies
- Medical Manager software
- Vista Care
- Vitalworks
- Web MD Intergy

2004 Mid-Year EMR Functionality Results

Based on our findings, the top thirteen EMR/EHR application vendors overall were:

Allscripts Healthcare Solutions, (TouchWorks EMR), www.TouchWorksEMR.com
Bond Technologies, www.bondclinician.com
Cerner Corporation, www.cerner.com
eClinicalWorks, www.eclinicalworks.com
Epic Systems, www.epicsystems.com
iMedica Corporation, www.imedica.com
InteGreat, www.iGreat.com
JMJ Technologies, Inc., www.jmjtech.com
Medical Communication Systems Inc., www.medcomsys.com
MedInformatix, Inc., www.medinformatix.com
NextGen Healthcare Information Systems, Inc., www.nextgen.com
Physician Micro Systems, www.pmsi.com
SynaMed, LLC, www.synamed.com

AC GROUP RELEASES 2004 MID YEAR EMR/EHR SURVEY
Extensive Evaluation Ranks Top EHR and EMR Applications

With the trend towards national standards and Pay-for-Performance guidelines, the mid-year functionality rating included 300 new questions that represented 18% of the point value ranking. The additional 300 questions challenged the vendors in ways that were never tested before.

EHR Functionality Ratings:

NextGen Healthcare Information Systems, Inc. continues to receive top honors in the annual EHR/EMR functionality report. With the acquisition of **Advanced Imaging Concepts**, the leading Healthcare specific Document Imaging Company, **Allscripts Healthcare Solutions** improved their overall functionality. Allscripts, Cerner[1], Epic and Nextgen were the only 4 vendors that received a 5-star rating this year in the EHR category.

Nine other vendors, Physician Micro System, Inc., SynaMed, JMJ Technologies, Medinformatics, InteGreat, Imedica Corporation, eClinicalWorks, Medical Communication Systems Inc, and Bond Technologies received 4-Star (80-89%) of required functionality. Eight others vendors received 3-Stars including, Cliniflow (Monarch), Vista Care, GE Medical Misys, Greenway, Vitalworks, MerianEMR, and Praxis (infor-med).

When evaluating vendor applications based on current and future functionality, five vendors are expected to increase their overall functionality and should be certified as a 5-star EHR application by the Spring of 2005. These top vendors include eClinicalworks, Bond Technologies, iMedica, Medical Communication Systems Inc, Physician Micro System, Inc., SynaMed, Medinformatics, and WebMD's Intergy product. Many of these vendors already meet the requirements of our EMR 5-star ranking; however, they do not meet all of the additional requirements to become a certified EHR application.

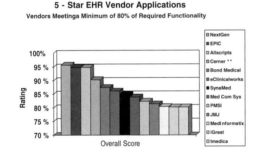

5 - Star EHR Vendor Applications
Vendors Meetinga Minimum of 80% of Required Functionality

Based on 4,583 Functional Questions Divided Between 27 Categories

---
[1] Cerner's self-reported rankings have not been tested as the time of this report.

AC GROUP RELEASES 2004 MID YEAR EMR/EHR SURVEY
Extensive Evaluation Ranks Top EHR and EMR Applications

EMR Functional Ratings - In many cases, physician practices are not interested in expanded EHR capabilities. Instead, they are evaluating vendors with strong EMR capability which may not included all of the national databases as in the EHR applications. The EMR products do include full charting system with automated E & M coding, drug alerts, limited national knowledgebase and clinical decision support, limited formulary compliance, summary of patient specific clinical results on one page. Additionally since the overall purchase price is usually 40% less, many physicians are satisfied with a certified EMR Application. The 5-Star rating EMR vendors are Bond Technologies, eClinicalworks, SynaMed, Med Communication Systems, PMSI, JMJ, MedInformatix, iGreat and Imedica. Of course all vendors that received a 4 or 5-star rating in the EHR category can also be considered in the EMR category. In all cases, the EHR vendors exceed the general requirements for an EMR.

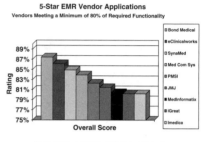

5-Star EMR Vendor Applications
Vendors Meeting a Minimum of 80% of Required Functionality

Based on 4,583 Functional Questions Divided Between 27 Categories

Charting System – The majority of the so-called EMR applications are really strong charting systems with complete clinical notes, limited alerts, limited clinical decision support, limited E & M coding methodology, and limited summary of patient clinical results on summary page. However, these systems still meet the needs of many physicians. The top vendors in the Charting System category include Cliniflow (Monarch), Vista Care, GE Medical, Misys, Greenway, Vitalworks, MerianEMR, Praxis (infor-med), Orion, A4 Healthcare, e-MDS, Chartcare, DR Notes, MDAnywhere, and McKesson.

Some of these vendors use standardized or customized templates while others allow more free-format charting. Once again, the EHR and EMR category vendors can also provide all of the needs of a base clinical charting system – but usually at a higher cost.

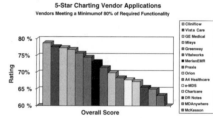

5-Star Charting Vendor Applications
Vendors Meeting a Minimum of 80% of Required Functionality

Based on 4,583 Functional Questions Divided Between 27 Categories

AC GROUP RELEASES 2004 MID YEAR EMR/EHR SURVEY
Extensive Evaluation Ranks Top EHR and EMR Applications

EMR Lite Application – The majority of the EMR applications are really strong EMR Lite systems with limited clinical note, e-prescribing, limited document image management, clinical results tracking and messaging, viewing of lab results and dictated reports. These systems are excellent for those physicians who elect to implement newer technologies in an incremental approach. These systems can assist a practice eliminate unnecessary tasks without changing the way a physician practices. Clinicians can view lab results and dictated reports from any location and can usually implement e-prescribing, along with medication, chief complaint, allergies, and vital signs tracking. The top EMR Lite application vendors include InteGreat, AIC Solutions, MedNet System, Axolotl, Healthvision, and Alteer.

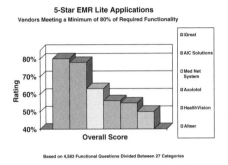

5-Star EMR Lite Applications
Vendors Meeting a Minimum of 80% of Required Functionality

Legend: iGreat, AIC Solutions, Med Net System, Axolotl, HealthVision, Alteer

Based on 4,583 Functional Questions Divided Between 27 Categories

Combined Practice Management, Document Imaging, and EMR/EHR products:

Although 94% of practices already have a practice management system (PMS), many physicians are considering the replacement of their older PMS with a new fully integrated or tightly interfaced PMS/DIM/EMR application. Many of the EMR vendors only offer and EMR and do not offer a PMS applications. The top vendor applications for a complete Digital Medical Office are:

Company	Updated Oct 2004	Updated May 2004	Updated Oct 2003	Desktop	EHR Rating	PMS Rating	Total Points
NextGen	Yes	Yes	Yes	95.6%	5	5	40
eClinicalworks	Yes	Yes	Yes	86.1%	4	4	29
SynaMed	Yes	Yes	Yes	84.9%	4	4	27
PMSI	Yes	Yes	Yes	82.3%	4	5	32
GE Medical	Yes	Yes	Yes	77.3%	3	5	34
Misys	Yes	Yes	Yes	76.8%	3	4	31
Greenway			Yes	75.7%	3	4	31
A4 Healthcare	Yes	Yes	Yes	68.4%	2	5	31
e-MDS			Yes	67.8%	2	4	27
McKesson	Yes	Yes	Yes	63.1%	2	5	36
Web MD Intergy	Yes	Yes	Yes	57.0%	1	5	37

NOTE: Ranking based on 5-Star system with 5 being the best. The Total points column takes into account each application, company viability, and end-user satisfaction.

AC GROUP RELEASES 2004 MID YEAR EMR/EHR SURVEY
Extensive Evaluation Ranks Top EHR and EMR Applications

Functionality is NOT the only Factor:

When evaluating companies, you must also take into account other factors such as, company size, company financial viability, total annual revenues, cash flow, % of revenue relating to EMR, EMR annual development costs, end-user satisfaction, number of employees, number of clients, cost per physician, and the company's ability to meet national, regional, and local standards. To assist, AC Group created a "point value" system that took these factors and others into account. Physicians should consider vendors with strong functionality ratings as well as "point value" ratings. The top EMR/EHR vendors for our mid-year 2004 report include:

- ○ NextGen
- ○ Allscripts
- ○ EPIC

- ○ GE Medical
- ○ Misys
- ○ PMSI

- ○ McKesson
- ○ A4 Healthcare
- ○ eClinicalworks

Actual Point Value Ratings:

Company	Updated Oct 2004	Updated May 2004	Updated Oct 2003	EHR Rating	EHR and Company Points
NextGen	Yes	Yes	Yes	95.6%	31
Allscripts	Yes	Yes	Yes	94.8%	31
EPIC	Yes	Yes	Yes	94.9%	30
GE Medical	Yes	Yes	Yes	77.3%	30
Misys	Yes	Yes	Yes	76.8%	28
PMSI	Yes	Yes	Yes	82.3%	27
McKesson	Yes	Yes	Yes	63.1%	27
A4 Healthcare	Yes	Yes	Yes	68.4%	26
eClinicalworks	Yes	Yes	Yes	86.1%	25
Vista Care		Yes	Yes	77.6%	24
Medical Manager		Yes	Yes	59.3%	23
JMJ	Yes	Yes	Yes	81.4%	22
iGreat	Yes	Yes	Yes	80.2%	22
Imedica	Yes	Yes	Yes	80.2%	22
Dr Notes		Yes	Yes	65.6%	22
Bond Medical	Yes	Yes	Yes	87.4%	21
MedInformatix		Yes	Yes	80.4%	21
e-MDS			Yes	67.8%	21
Medinotes	Yes	Yes	Yes	59.5%	21
Web MD Intergy	Yes	Yes	Yes	57.0%	21
Cerner **	Yes	Yes	Yes	90.3%	20
Praxis (infor-med)	Yes	Yes	Yes	71.4%	20
SynaMed	Yes	Yes	Yes	84.9%	19
Med Com Sys	Yes	Yes	Yes	83.9%	19
Vitalworks			Yes	74.5%	19
Axolotl	Yes	Yes	Yes	56.2%	19

AC GROUP RELEASES 2004 MID YEAR EMR/EHR SURVEY
Extensive Evaluation Ranks Top EHR and EMR Applications

Size Does Matter:

Rating vendors only on functionality is not always helpful since certain vendors only sell their products to specific market demographics. For example, of the 44 vendor applications evaluated, 12 sell to smaller physician offices with 1-4 physicians, and only 10 sell to practices with more than 100 physicians. To help physicians understand which vendors are best for them, we have attempted to divide the marketplace based on practice size. Additionally, practices should require the vendors to provide them with references from practices of similar size and similar specialty. However, just because a vendor does NOT have similar sized references does not necessary mean that they cannot technically meet your requirements, It may however mean that your practice size or specialty is new to the vendor. In those cases, we recommend negotiating a lower overall product price,

Ranking	Company	EHR Rating	Total Points	Number of Providers in the Practice					
				1 to 5	6 to 15	16 - 49	49 - 99	100 to 249	> 250
1	NextGen	95.6%	31		Yes	Yes	Yes	Yes	Yes
2	EPIC	94.9%	30					Yes	Yes
3	Allscripts	94.8%	31		Yes	Yes	Yes	Yes	Yes
4	Cerner **	90.3%	20				Yes	Yes	Yes
5	Bond Medical	87.4%	21	Yes	Yes	Yes	Yes		
6	eClinicalworks	86.1%	25	Yes	Yes	Yes	Yes	Yes	
7	SynaMed	84.9%	19	Yes	Yes	Yes	Yes	Yes	Yes
8	Med Com Sys	83.9%	19		Yes	Yes	Yes	Yes	Yes
9	PMSI	82.3%	27	Yes	Yes	Yes	Yes	Yes	Yes
10	JMJ	81.4%	22	Yes	Yes				
11	MedInformatix	80.4%	21	Yes	Yes	Yes	Yes		
12	iGreat	80.2%	22				Yes	Yes	Yes
13	Imedica	80.2%	22		Yes	Yes	Yes	Yes	Yes

AC GROUP RELEASES 2004 MID YEAR EMR/EHR SURVEY
Extensive Evaluation Ranks Top EHR and EMR Applications

Large Practices (> 100 Physicians) - For larger practices with over 150 physicians, the top applications are from NextGen Healthcare Systems (95.6%), Allscripts Healthcare Solutions (94.8%), and Epic (94.9%). Allscripts is the 2004 TEPR award winner for large EMR Applications and Nextgen was the TEPR award winner in 2001-04 and the MSHUG award winner in 2003 and 2004. Cerner received a 90.3% rating but have not been certified at the time of this report. Five additional vendors, iMedica Corporation, McKesson, and GE Medical scored high EHR functionality rating. NextGen, Allscripts and Epic received the highest overall point ranking once you consider company size, client base, end-user satisfaction, and price. Given the resent trends towards community systems, Regional Health Information Organizations, and Pay-for-Performance, larger practices should look towards those vendors with 3-5 star ratings in the EHR category only.

	Company	City	State	Desktop	Rating	Total Points
1	NextGen	Horsham	PA	95.6%	5.00	32
2	EPIC	Madison	WI	94.9%	5.00	30
3	Allscripts	Libertyville	IL	94.8%	5.00	32
4	Cerner **	Kansas City	MO	90.3%	5.00	20
5	Imedica	Mountain View	CA	80.2%	4.00	22
6	GE Medical	Milwaukee	WI	77.3%	3.00	30
7	Misys	Tucson	AZ	76.8%	3.00	28
8	McKesson	Alpharetta	GA	63.1%	3.00	27

Top EMR/EHR Vendor Applications

Large Practices > 100 Physicians

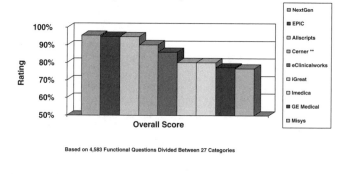

Based on 4,583 Functional Questions Divided Between 27 Categories

AC GROUP RELEASES 2004 MID YEAR EMR/EHR SURVEY
Extensive Evaluation Ranks Top EHR and EMR Applications

Mid Size Practices (9 to 99 Physicians)

For larger practices with between 9 and 99 physicians, the top applications are from NextGen Healthcare Systems (95.6%) and Allscripts Healthcare Solutions (94.8%). Six additional vendors, Bond Technologies (87.4%), eClinicalworks (86.1%), SynaMed (84.9%), Medical Communication Systems (83.9%), Physician Micro Systems (82.3%), JMJ (81.4%) and Medinformatics (80.4%), and scored 5-Stars in the EMR functionality rating. Meridian EMR, Misys, Greenway, Praxis, and GE Medical received 3-Stars. NextGen and Allscripts received the highest overall point ranking once you consider company size, client base, end-user satisfaction, and price.

	Company	City	State	Desktop	EHR Rating	EMR Rating	Total Points
1	NextGen	Horsham	PA	97.1%	5.00	5.00	32
2	Allscripts	Libertyville	IL	92.9%	5.00	5.00	32
3	Bond Tech	Tampa	FL	87.4%	4.0	5.00	21
4	eClinicalworks	Northboro	MA	86.1%	4.00	5.00	25
5	SynaMed	Kew Gardens	NY	84.9%	4.00	5.00	19
6	Medical Comm. Systems, Inc.	Woburn	MA	83.9%	4.00	5.00	19
7	PMSI	Seattle	WA	82.3%	4.00	5.00	27
8	MedInformatix	Los Angles	CA	80.4%	4.00	5.00	21

Top EMR/EHR Vendor Applications

Mid –Sized Practices from 9 to 99 Physicians

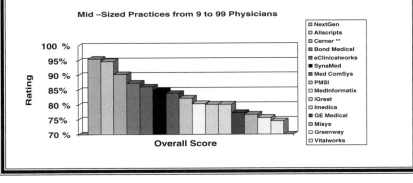

AC GROUP RELEASES 2004 MID YEAR EMR/EHR SURVEY
Extensive Evaluation Ranks Top EHR and EMR Applications

Small Practices - (5 – 9 Physicians)

For smaller practices with 5 to 9 physicians, once again, the top applications remain the same as the mid-sized practices.   Two new vendors entered this category – Bond Technologies (88.1%) and JMJ Technologies (79.0%). In most cases, many of these vendors do not actively market to the size of practice. However, all will provide a bid if requested.

	Company	City	State	Desktop	Last Updated˙	EMR Rating	Total Points
1	Bond Tech	Tampa	FL	87.4%	Oct 2004	5	21
2	eClinicalworks	Northboro	MA	86.1%	Oct 2004	5	25
3	SynaMed	Kew Gardens	NY	84.9%	Oct 2004	5	19
4	Medical Comm. Systems, Inc.	Woburn	MA	83.9%	Oct 2004	5	19
5	PMSI	Seattle	WA	82.3%	Oct 2004	5	27
6	JMJ	Marietta	GA	81.4%	Oct 2004	5	22
7	MedInformatix	Los Angeles	CA	80.4%	May 2004	5	21
8	Misys	Tucson	AZ	76.8%	Oct 2004	4	28
9	Greenway	Carrollton	GA	75.7%	2003	4	18
10	MeridianEMR		NJ	73.2%	Oct 2004	4	14
11	A4 Healthcare	Cary	NC	68.4%	Oct 2004	3	26
12	e-MDS	Cedar Park	TX	67.8%	2003	3	21

AC GROUP RELEASES 2004 MID YEAR EMR/EHR SURVEY
Extensive Evaluation Ranks Top EHR and EMR Applications

Small Practices - (1 – 4 Physicians)

For smaller practices with less than 5 physicians that are satisfied with an EMR application, **SynaMed, Bond Technologies, Physician Micro Systems, and eClinicalworks** received 5 Stars in EMR ratings with more than 80% of the current requirements. **Physician Micro Systems** and eClinicalworks received the highest overall point ranking once you consider company size, client base, end-user satisfaction, and price. PraxisEMR, JMJ Technologies, Meridian EMR, MedInformatix, A4 Healthcare, and Greenway Medical rounded out the top 10 EMR vendor applications for the small physician office. The rating by vendor is displayed below:

	Company	City	State	Desktop	Last Updated˙	EMR Rating	Total Points
1	Bond Tech	Tampa	FL	87.4%	Oct 2004	5	21
2	eClinicalworks	Northboro	MA	86.1%	Oct 2004	5	25
3	SynaMed	Kew Gardens	NY	84.9%	Oct 2004	5	19
4	Medical Comm. Systems, Inc.	Woburn	MA	83.9%	Oct 2004	5	19
5	PMSI	Seattle	WA	82.3%	Oct 2004	5	27
6	JMJ	Marietta	GA	81.4%	Oct 2004	5	22
7	MedInformatix	Los Angeles	CA	80.4%	May 2004	5	21
8	MeridianEMR		NJ	73.2%	Oct 2004	4	14
9	PraxisEMR	Woodland Hills	CA	71.4%	Oct 2004	4	20
10	A4 Healthcare	Cary	NC	68.4%	Oct 2004	3	26
11	e-MDS	Cedar Park	TX	67.8%	2003	3	21

AC GROUP RELEASES 2004 MID YEAR EMR/EHR SURVEY
Extensive Evaluation Ranks Top EHR and EMR Applications

Conclusion:

Technology is only a tool and if used effectively can improve the flow of information and potentially improve the efficiency of the physician's practice. However in reality, if "change" is not embraced, the probability of success is very low. We learned in the 1980's that we needed to change the process of billing for services – or we would not be paid in a timely and effective manner. Therefore, the practice of medicine, from the business point of view, changed. Now with newer technologies, government regulations, and the right financial incentive, physicians will begin embracing new levels of technology that were not available just 5 years ago. But where does a physician in a small practice turn to learn about the 100's of technology choices? The physician can spend hours searching and evaluating all of the opportunities. Or maybe in the near future, physicians will be able to look towards leaders within their own medical specialty for guidance and knowledge.

More about the Author:

Mark R. Anderson, FHIMSS, CPHIMS – Healthcare IT Futurist

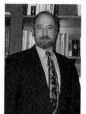

Mr. Anderson is one of the nation's premier IT research futurists dedicated to health care. He is one of the leading national speakers on healthcare and physician practices and has spoken at > 350 conferences and meetings since 2000. He has spent the last 32+ years focusing on Healthcare – not just technology questions, but strategic, policy, and organizational considerations. He tracks industry trends, conducts member surveys and case studies, assesses best practices, and performs benchmarking studies.

Mr. Anderson is also the CIO for the Taconic IPA, a 2,300 Physician IPA based in upper New York. Prior to forming AC Group, Inc. in February of 2000, Mr. Anderson was the worldwide head and VP of healthcare for META Group, Inc., the Chief Information Officer (CIO) with West Tennessee Healthcare, the Corporate CIO for the Sisters of Charity of Nazareth Health System, the Corporate Internal IT Consultant with the Sisters of Providence (SOP) Hospitals, and the Executive Director for Management Services for Denver Health and Hospitals and Harris County Hospital District.

His experience **includes 22+ years working with physician offices, 9 years in the development of physician-based MSO's,** 17 years with multi-facility Health Care organizations, 15 years Administrative Executive Team experience, 6 years as a member of the Corporate Executive Team, and 9 years in healthcare turnaround consulting. Mr. Anderson received his BS in Business, is completing his MBA in Health Care Administration, and is a Certified Fellow with HIMSS.

E-Mail: mra@acgroup.org

Operating in a Vacuum: *New York Times* Editorial

May 3, 2004

Operating in a Vacuum

By Newt Gingrich and Patrick Kennedy

WASHINGTON—Health care policy is a partisan minefield, with Democrats and Republicans differing on everything from Medicare changes to malpractice reform to strategies for covering the uninsured. Yet, while the two of us have been on opposite sides of most of those battles, we both believe that America's health care delivery system must be transformed. To begin that transformation, we should heed President Bush's call last week for widespread adoption of electronic health records. As the president noted, "The 21st-century health care system is using a 19th-century paperwork system."

The archaic information systems of our hospitals and clinics directly affect the quality of care we receive. When you go to a new doctor, the office most likely has little information about you, no ability to track how other providers are treating you, and no systematic way to keep up with scientific breakthroughs that might help you.

The results are predictable. For example, approximately 20 percent of medical tests are ordered a second time simply because previous results can't be found. Research shows that 30 cents of every dollar spent on health care does nothing to make sick people better. That's $7.4 trillion over the next decade for duplicate tests, preventable errors, unnecessary hospitalizations and other waste.

Not only do these unnecessary costs contribute to skyrocketing insurance premiums, but the lack of good information makes improvements in quality and efficiency nearly impossible. Every year some 98,000 Americans die in the hospital from preventable medical errors, like receiving the wrong medication. Nearly half of patients do not get all the treatments or tests that should have been administered. This is usually not the fault of doctors, nurses and other health professionals—these problems persist because of systemic failures stemming from the absence of good health information.

The problem is not that we need innovation: existing technology can transform health care just as it has nearly every other part of society. If all Americans' electronic health records were connected in secure computer networks that safeguarded patient privacy, health care providers would have complete records for their patients, so they would no longer have to re-order tests that have already been done.

In addition, most referrals and prescriptions are still written by hand; computerized entry would eliminate errors caused by sloppy handwriting. Computer programs can warn doctors of possible adverse drug and allergy interactions, and remind them of new advances in evidence-based practice guidelines. Patients could also have easier access to their important health information, allowing them to be active participants in their own care.

Moreover, in a post-9/11 world, electronic health information networks would allow doctors, hospitals and public health officials to rapidly detect and respond to a bioterrorism attack.

Unfortunately, health care providers are famously stingy investors in information technology. The primary reason is that when new technology reduces the duplication, errors and unnecessary care, most of the financial benefits don't go to the providers who generate the savings, but to insurers and patients.

Therefore, widespread adoption of technology will depend in large part on federally organized public-private partnerships. Treasury dollars could help bring providers in a particular part of the country together to map out plans for a regional health information network, and to divide up the costs and the savings fairly between them. Medicare could sweeten the pot by reimbursing providers for money spent to use electronic health records connected to a regional network.

New information systems would also allow us to reinvent the way providers get paid. Right now, most doctors and hospitals get paid by the procedure, regardless of quality. They get paid even if they make mistakes, and then paid again to fix the mistakes. And under our current perverse payment practices, when providers improve quality and efficiency, it frequently hurts their bottom lines.

New information systems would give us nationwide data to develop standardized performance measurements for providers, so anybody can get an apples-to-apples comparison about how good a job a doctor or hospital does. This data would also allow Medicare and private plans to restructure their reimbursement practices, so that the market would drive competition in quality and value among hospitals and doctors, just as in most other fields.

Politicians like to say that the United States has the best health care system in the world. Actually, what we have right now is the best medical talent, technology and facilities in the world—but the system that delivers our care is badly broken. Democrats and Republicans should agree that moving American medicine into the 21st century is not only an important goal, it is also literally a matter of life and death.

Newt Gingrich, a former Republican speaker of the House, is the founder of the Center for Health Transformation, a for-profit organization. Patrick J. Kennedy, a Democrat, is a representative from Rhode Island.

Reproduced with permission from the *New York Times.*

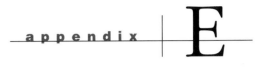
Test Your Knowledge of EMR/EHR Implementation

The following quiz can help to test your knowledge of electronic medical record (EMR) and electronic health record (EHR) implementation. Circle the correct letter and then check your answers with the answer key at the end.

1. The Institute of Medicine published what document that helped shape the business and quality of healthcare for patients, healthcare organizations, policy officials, and healthcare workers?

   a) *Saving Lives & Saving Money* by Newt Gingrich

   b) The Medicare Modernization Act of 2003

   c) Health Insurance Portability and Accountability Act of 1996

   d) *Crossing the Quality Chasm: A New Health System for the 21st Century*

2. Former Secretary of Health and Human Services, Tommy Thompson, referred to the "Decade of Health Information Technology" as what period of time?

   a) 1996–2006, when HIPAA's Privacy, Security, and Transactions and Code Sets Rules are implemented

   b) 2010–2020, when Baby Boomers begin to apply for Medicare

   c) 2020–2030, when GenXers begin to pay down the national debt

   d) 2004–2014, when the government shifts its policy focus from administrative to clinical standards

3. The federal agency established by President George W. Bush to roll out the national health information technology (HIT) plan is:

   a) The Agency for Health Research and Quality

   b) The Office of the National Coordinator for Health Information Technology

   c) The Department of Homeland Security

   d) The US Department of Health and Human Services

4. The move to health information technology is likely to change the way physicians practice medicine.
    a) True
    b) False

5. Key audiences involved in the move to health information technology include:
    a) Physicians
    b) Hospitals and academic medical centers
    c) Patients
    d) All of the above

6. The patient version of the EHR is often called:
    a) An automated teller machine
    b) A handheld computer
    c) A Personal Health Record
    d) A debit card

7. EHRs are patient focused.
    a) True
    b) False

8. EMRs are physician focused.
    a) True
    b) False

9. To understand what will change in the move to technology, you should:
    a) Evaluate and map your workflow
    b) Engage the EHR implementation team
    c) Establish a budget for an EHR implementation
    d) All of the above

10. You probably want an EHR system that:
    a) Saves time and improves cash flow
    b) Improves patient safety
    c) Provides up-to-date clinical information
    d) All of the above

11. When you prioritize your EHR system functions, you:
    a) Annoy the EMR vendor
    b) Make smarter decisions and achieve outcomes

c) Delegate the selection responsibility to your best employee

d) Have no fear about EHR implementation

12. EHR Certification will:

a) Reduce the risk of information technology (IT) investment

b) Improve the functioning of the IT marketplace

c) Facilitate IT adoption incentives by payers and purchasers

d) All of the above

13. Before purchasing the EMR/EHR system, you should:

a) Establish an implementation dream team

b) Prioritize functions and existing system capabilities

c) Submit an RFP to several vendors and rate their responses on a scorecard

d) All of the above

14. Interoperability means:

a) The ability to perform a surgical procedure in multiple locations

b) The ability to speak more than one language

c) The ability to exchange and use information

d) The ability to connect several telephone systems into one network

15. When negotiating an EHR, which is the most important element you must protect:

a) Your hardware systems

b) Your patient's attitudes about your EHR system

c) Your relationship with the vendor

d) Your data

16. The federal government's Consolidated Health Informatics Initiative (CHI) only impacts directly federal government health-related programs, agencies, and departments.

a) True

b) False

17. The foundation of the CHI initiative is to use the same clinical vocabularies (code sets) and the same ways of transmitting that information.

a) True

b) False

18. The private healthcare sector is off the hook with respect to the clinical standards adopted by the federal government.

    a) True—this is a federal initiative and will impact only those in government health-related programs

    b) False—the federal government is leading by example and using its considerable size in the US healthcare sector to encourage adoption of the same clinical standards

19. The Institute of Medicine designed a model of an EHR system and requested Health Level Seven (HL7) to produce a draft standard for trial use. What is the physician's role in this process?

    a) Review the standards and make comments on what you like or do not like

    b) Stay out of the way and let them do their work

    c) Write his or her congressional representative

    d) Find work elsewhere

20. Refocusing healthcare around the consumer by implementing health information technology can improve quality of care, patient safety and physician efficiency.

    a) True

    b) False

ANSWER KEY

1. D	11. B
2. D	12. D
3. B	13. D
4. A	14. C
5. D	15. D
6. C	16. A
7. A	17. A
8. A	18. B
9. D	19. A
10. D	20. A

INDEX